THE
POWER
VISION
PROGRAM
FOR
BETTER
EYESIGHT

THE
POWER
VISION
PROGRAM

FOR

BETTER
EYESIGHT

CLINICALLY PROVEN
NATURAL METHOD TO
SEE MORE CLEARLY
IN 30 DAYS OR LESS

VISION THERAPY ASSOCIATES ⚕

MERRILL J. ALLEN, O.D., PH.D. | STEVEN M. BERESFORD, PH.D. | FRANCIS A. YOUNG, PH.D.

Humanix Books
www.humanixbooks.com

Humanix Books

THE POWER VISION PROGRAM FOR BETTER EYESIGHT

Copyright © 2025 by Humanix Books

All rights reserved.

Humanix Books, P.O. Box 20989, West Palm Beach, FL 33416, USA

www.humanixbooks.com | info@humanixbooks.com

Humanix Books is a division of Humanix Publishing, LLC. Its trademark, consisting of the words "Humanix Books," is registered in the United States Patent and Trademark Office and in other countries.

Humanix Books titles may be purchased for educational, business, or sales promotional use. For information about special discounts for bulk purchases, please contact the Special Markets Department at info@humanixbooks.com.

Cover image by iStock/Phillip Steury

Back cover image by Shutterstock/Irina Bg

Disclaimer: The information presented in this book is not specific medical advice for any individual and should not substitute medical advice from a health professional. If you have (or think you may have) a medical problem, speak to your doctor or a health professional immediately about your risk and treatments. Do not engage in any care of treatment without consulting a medical professional.

ISBN: 978-163006-322-1 (Paperback)

ISBN: 978-163006-323-8 (E-book)

Printed in the United States of America

10 9 8 7 6 5 4 3 2 1

CONTENTS

INTRODUCING THE POWER VISION PROGRAM

Meet the Authors

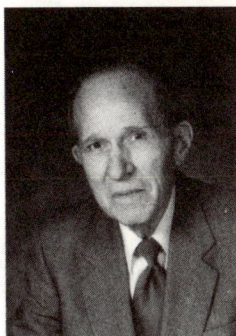

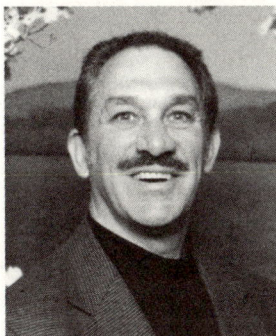

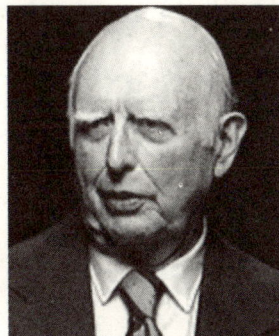

Dr. Merrill J. Allen, O.D., Ph.D.

Former Head of the Optometry School at Indiana University. During his distinguished career, he educated thousands of optometrists and published 236 research papers. He received 21 professional honors including the American Optometric Association's prestigious Apollo Award and the British Optical Association's Research Medal.

Dr. Steven M. Beresford, Ph.D.

Research scientist who was pivotal in maximizing the effectiveness of the techniques in the Power Vision Program. He has carried out extensive research into the biomechanics of the eyes, including cataract reversal.

Dr. Francis A. Young, Ph.D.

Former Head of Washington State University Primate Research Center. He published 120 research papers and received 11 honors including the American Optometric Association's Apollo Award for his myopia research.

SECTION

1

THE
VISION
THERAPY
ALTERNATIVE

Like most people with poor vision, you probably believe your condition is hopeless and there's nothing you can do except rely on stronger glasses every few years as your eyesight gets worse, followed by a disease such as cataracts or macular degeneration.

Fortunately, there's a better way.

An elite group of eye care professionals known as *behavioral optometrists* have developed dozens of effective *vision therapy eye exercises*. These enhance the performance of the entire visual system, resulting in healthier, more relaxed eyes, naturally better eyesight, and a more satisfying lifestyle.

The Power Vision Program gives you the best of these exercises.

If you've resigned yourself to a lifetime of inferior vision, there's a new day dawning. A new freedom you never thought possible. A clearer, brighter future is only a few short weeks away! Follow the Power Vision Program as directed, and you can expect to:

- Get healthier eyes with more natural focusing ability

- Avoid or reduce dependency on corrective lenses

- Improve dry eyes and sensitivity to bright light

- Get relief from computer eyestrain and headaches

- Have faster reading and better comprehension

- Lower the risk of degenerative eye diseases

- Reduce wrinkles around the eyes

As you read the Power Vision Program, you'll learn many new words and concepts. Don't worry that it's too complicated. The knowledge you're about to gain can keep your eyes strong and healthy into old age and reduce the risk of potentially blinding eye diseases, so persevere and don't give up!

Simply follow the directions and learn the exercises, and everything will soon fall into place. We recommend reading each section three times so that you get a good understanding of the contents, or at least understand the main points.

The Power Vision Program is based on the latest scientific and clinical research and can reliably produce the following results:

Group One: If your eyesight is starting to go bad and you think you need glasses, or you're wearing your first pair of glasses, the Power Vision Program can probably help you return to normal within a few weeks.

Group Two: If you've worn glasses for more than a year and your eyesight is getting worse, the Power Vision Program can probably reverse the deterioration within a few weeks and help you avoid a stronger prescription.

Group Three: If you've worn glasses for more than a year and you want to reduce your dependency on them or get rid of them altogether, the Power Vision Program can probably help you. It usually takes two or three months to get the maximum amount of improvement.

Clinically Tested Eye Exercises

The Power Vision Program provides you with 16 clinically tested eye exercises, divided into three modules.

The first module—the **Power Exercises**—forms the dynamic core of the program and will give your entire visual system a good basic tune-up, like tuning up an engine. You will feel positive changes taking place in your eyes within a few days and will see the first signs of improvement in a week or so.

The second module—the **Booster Exercises**—is a set of stress reduction techniques that will make your eyes feel wonderfully invigorated and relaxed.

The third module—the **Fusion Exercises**—builds on the results obtained from the Power Exercises and will increase the range and flexibility of your focusing system.

Spend at least 10 minutes a day doing as many of the exercises as possible. Don't overdo it or strain your eyes, but the more you do, the more improvement you'll get and the sooner you'll get it.

The Power Vision Program can give you really fast results. We advise you to start doing the exercises today. Don't procrastinate. Don't wait or make excuses. Follow the Seven Steps to Success, and cultivate the habit of doing one or more exercise modules per day.

Seven Steps to Success

Step 1: Skim through the entire Power Vision Program. Don't spend more than a couple of minutes on this. All you need is a general idea of the material so you know what to expect. Read the entire Power Vision Program when you have enough time.

Step 2: Decide what your goal is. Is your vision starting to go bad and you want to avoid glasses? Do you already wear glasses and want to avoid a stronger prescription? Do you already wear glasses and want to reduce your dependency on them or get rid of them altogether?

Step 3: Read the entire Power Exercise module. Some of the exercises will become your New Visual Habits. The goal is to do them during some of your daily activities so they become part of your lifestyle. Start doing them today.

Step 4: Make several copies of the Progress Report (Section 1), Reminder Card (Section 1), and Biofeedback Charts (Section 3). Put the Reminder Card in prominent positions in your home, workspace, and car. Use the Biofeedback Charts as targets for Flexing and Detailing.

Step 5: Set up a special place to do the exercises, preferably a blank section of wall with good lighting and a table to put things on. Set an alarm clock for the time you will do your daily exercise session. Using an alarm clock is the best way to remind yourself to do the exercises, so do this now before you get sidetracked and forget!

Step 6: Start doing the Power Exercises. Read the instructions carefully and make sure you're doing them correctly. Don't rush. Speed is not important. Aim for control and good coordination. Cultivate the habit of exercising your eyes on a regular basis, even if it's just 10 minutes a day, and you'll soon get results!

Step 7: Identify and understand your visual problem. Read Section 8. Are you nearsighted, farsighted, or presbyopic? Do you have astigmatism or a lazy eye? Section 8 will give you a good understanding of your visual problem together with advice and therapy techniques. Get an eye exam to make sure you don't have anything wrong with your eyes that requires specialized care.

Your New Visual Habits

Most of our actions, including the operation of the visual system, are controlled by habit patterns that help us do ordinary things without having to constantly make decisions. Instead of wasting time and energy consciously calculating every action, we rely on habit patterns to help us live normally without really thinking about what we're doing.

Behavioral optometrists have found that most people with poor vision have negative visual habits such as bad posture, reading or doing close work without taking a break, and leaving their glasses on all the time. By endlessly repeating negative visual habits, the eyeball may eventually go out of shape.

Improving your vision means getting rid of negative visual habits and replacing them with positive ones. These will make ordinary activities and objects more interesting, and you'll develop a better way of looking at the world—a brighter, clearer way of seeing!

Your success depends on diligently cultivating the habit of doing the exercises on a daily basis until they are part of your lifestyle. It takes about a month to establish a new habit, so use an alarm clock and the Progress Report (Section 1) to keep you on track.

In addition to doing the exercise modules, six of the exercises (Blinking, Clocking, Detailing, Flexing, Pushups, and Rolling) enable you to do vision therapy during some of your normal activities without taking up any extra time. These are your New Visual Habits, and you can even do them in a room full of people without anyone realizing what you're doing!

Your goal is to convert *dead time*, when you aren't doing anything in particular, into vision therapy. There are three major periods of dead time: stopping at traffic lights, during TV and YouTube commercials, and standing in line at stores and restaurants.

You must resolutely integrate your New Visual Habits with these events. You must resolutely do the exercises until they become part of your normal way of waiting at traffic lights, during TV and YouTube commercials, and standing in line. The beauty of this strategy is that it doesn't take up any extra time. You're simply using your time more efficiently and living your life more productively!

> **Your goal is to convert *dead time*, when you aren't doing anything in particular, into vision therapy.**

Do Vision Therapy at Traffic Lights

The time spent waiting at traffic lights provides most people with the best opportunity for everyday practice. If you live in a city, you probably stop at about 10 traffic lights a day and spend a minute or two at each light. If you stay at home most of the time, TV and YouTube commercials provide the best opportunity, which you can use in addition to traffic lights.

This can add up to 15 minutes a day of dead time where you're stuck in your car and there's no escape. You can't avoid traffic lights, and they're only going to become more numerous as the city expands. So what are you going to do? Pound your fists on the steering wheel and drive yourself into a frenzied fit of anger and frustration?

Not anymore! From this day forth, practice your New Visual Habits every time you stop at a traffic light until they become part of your normal driving routine. Tape a Reminder Card and a Biofeedback chart to the dashboard. Do one or more exercises at each light.

Same goes for TV and YouTube commercials and standing in line. Tape a Reminder Card and a Biofeedback chart to your computer, TV, or somewhere in your workspace. Develop the habit of exercising your eyes during these periods of dead time. Even if it's just doing some Blinking or Clocking or Detailing, the exercises will work together to give you healthier eyes and a lifetime of naturally better eyesight!

> **You can do the exercises without understanding how your eyes work, in which case read Section 2 later.**

Progress Report

Date _____

	M	T	W	T	F	S	S
Clocking	☐	☐	☐	☐	☐	☐	☐
Flexing	☐	☐	☐	☐	☐	☐	☐
Blinking	☐	☐	☐	☐	☐	☐	☐
Pushups	☐	☐	☐	☐	☐	☐	☐
Rolling	☐	☐	☐	☐	☐	☐	☐
Detailing	☐	☐	☐	☐	☐	☐	☐
Conducting	☐	☐	☐	☐	☐	☐	☐
Biofeedback	☐	☐	☐	☐	☐	☐	☐
Hydrotherapy	☐	☐	☐	☐	☐	☐	☐
Palming	☐	☐	☐	☐	☐	☐	☐
Light Therapy	☐	☐	☐	☐	☐	☐	☐
Acupressure	☐	☐	☐	☐	☐	☐	☐
Eccentric Circles	☐	☐	☐	☐	☐	☐	☐
Fusion Chart	☐	☐	☐	☐	☐	☐	☐
Fusion Flexing	☐	☐	☐	☐	☐	☐	☐
Thumb Fusion	☐	☐	☐	☐	☐	☐	☐

Comments: _____

VISION
THERAPY
ASSOCIATES

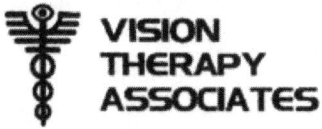

REMINDER CARD

ROLLING
FLEXING
PUSHUPS
BLINKING
CLOCKING
DETAILING

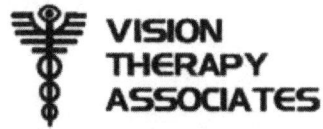

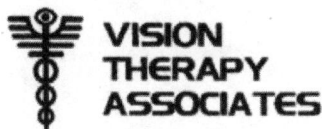

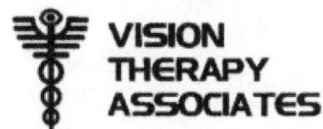

VISION
THERAPY
ASSOCIATES

REMINDER CARD

ROLLING
FLEXING
PUSHUPS
BLINKING
CLOCKING
DETAILING

VISION
THERAPY
ASSOCIATES

REMINDER CARD

ROLLING
FLEXING
PUSHUPS
BLINKING
CLOCKING
DETAILING

VISION
THERAPY
ASSOCIATES

REMINDER CARD

ROLLING
FLEXING
PUSHUPS
BLINKING
CLOCKING
DETAILING

SECTION

(2)

WELCOME TO THE POWER VISION PROGRAM

Good Vision Is Your Birthright

The explosive growth of alternative health care is more than a fad. It reflects a widespread dissatisfaction with the status quo. Millions of health-conscious people are fed up with old, ineffective treatment procedures and are looking for better, safer, more natural methods of healing.

Like most people with bad eyesight, you've probably been told that you can't cure or improve your visual problem—or even stop it from getting worse—and there's nothing you can do except resign yourself to a lifetime of progressively stronger corrective lenses followed by drugs or surgery if you develop an eye disease.

Nothing could be further from the truth.

A wide range of vision therapy eye exercises are now available that will make your eyes healthier and improve your focusing power naturally. In many cases, the exercises reduce or eliminate the need for corrective lenses.

Many people find vision therapy to be an interesting and stimulating form of self-improvement, like learning how to ride a bicycle or play a musical instrument. Learning the different exercises can be a fascinating and rewarding experience that will benefit you for the rest of your life.

Realize that you are now entering an important period of personal development. Instead of helplessly watching your eyesight get worse, you can now do something positive about it. So don't be lazy. Don't let this opportunity slip through your fingers. The Power Vision Program gives you the opportunity to enjoy a lifetime of healthier eyes and better vision. Take advantage of it.

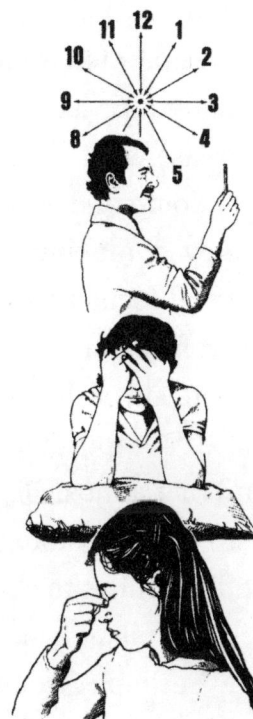

You are about to gain a lot of important information about your eyes based on the latest clinical and scientific research. Knowledge is power, and although you can do the exercises without a deep understanding of how your eyes work, we advise you to learn the basic principles.

Tuning Up Your Visual System

The Power Vision Program gives your eyes a good basic workout, like tuning up an engine. In contrast to physical exercises, however, eye exercises are not strenuous. They work by increasing the range and accuracy of the ciliary muscles, extraocular muscles, and other functions of the visual system. They don't make the eye muscles bigger or stronger.

The Power Vision Program will stretch, tone, and condition the muscles in and around your eyes, making them operate beyond their normal range of activity. It will make your visual system more flexible and dynamic and increase what are known as *degrees of freedom*.

Some of the exercises stimulate the flow of nutrients to the eyes, making them healthier. Other exercises increase natural focusing power and reduce eyestrain from reading or working at a computer. Other exercises reverse or delay the effects of the aging process.

> **Almost all cases of poor vision begin with nothing more serious than a minor focusing error.**

It's important to understand that about 98% of babies have normal, healthy eyes, and that almost all young children have good vision. Almost all cases of poor vision begin with nothing more serious than a minor focusing error. This is a very important concept, and it applies to children, teenagers, and adults, so please take a moment to think about it and let it sink in.

Perhaps distant objects have become slightly blurred, or you now find it difficult to read a menu. Perhaps your eyes get tired from working at a computer or playing video games. The point is that nobody goes to bed with normal, healthy vision and wakes up the next morning with deformed eyeballs!

The Genetic Theory of Poor Vision

The traditional method of treatment with corrective lenses is based on the theory that most visual problems are caused by genetic deformities, like a cleft palate or a clubbed foot. This theory has never been proved, and the majority of behavioral optometrists believe that it should be modified or abandoned altogether.

Our research, together with that of other scientists and eye care professionals, has shown that nearsightedness (myopia) is usually caused by watching TV too close, doing too much reading, or staring at a computer or smartphone. In general, looking at near objects for long periods of time causes *nearpoint stress*, which increases the pressure inside the eyeball and gradually makes it go out of shape and become elongated.

Bankrupting the Genetic Theory

Since almost everyone is born with normal, healthy eyes, what the genetic theory proposes is that millions of normal, healthy children are mysteriously mutating into adults with genetically deformed eyeballs. There's no precedent whatsoever for such a bizarre phenomenon. Normal, healthy children never develop cleft palates or clubfeet, and there's no reason to suppose that the eyeballs are an exception to this rule.

Can you imagine the panic that would ensue if millions of normal, healthy children started mutating into adults with clubfeet? Do you think they would be satisfied if doctors blamed it on genetics and said that apart from surgery, nothing could be done except wear special shoes for the rest of their lives, and they would need larger sizes every few years as the problem got worse? The scenario is so absurd that it hardly bears consideration.

The predictions made by the genetic theory also fail to pass the test. If vision is genetic in origin, it shouldn't change after the person grows up, because the shape and size of the eyeball are determined by the bone structure of the eye socket, which is immutable in adults.

However, since the widespread use of computers, millions of adults with normal, healthy vision develop myopia after the age of 30, which is long after the body stops growing. This and other examples have demolished the credibility of the genetic theory. Scientists and behavioral optometrists who are familiar with the evidence regard the genetic theory as incorrect and intellectually bankrupt.

Use It or Lose It

A similar situation exists with regard to presbyopia, which is part of the aging process and affects everyone. There's no escape. You can run but you can't hide. Sooner or later, presbyopia takes its toll. Therein lies an important point. Later is better than sooner.

Previous generations were doomed to suffer the "whips and scorns of time"—the aches and pains of growing old, losing their health, strength, and mental abilities as they awaited the arrival of the Grim Reaper. Nowadays, we have the knowledge and power to delay his arrival.

By making a few simple changes in our lifestyle, we can grow old gracefully.

One of the most exciting discoveries of the twentieth century is that by making a few simple changes in our lifestyle, we can grow old gracefully instead of becoming senile and decrepit. Many people now realize that aging is a "use it or lose it" situation, and by staying physically active, they can maintain good health much longer than was previously thought possible. This principle also applies to the eyes.

Almost all common visual problems can be improved with the exercises you are about to learn. However, the Power Vision Program is not a "throw away your glasses" system. Although some people get amazing results, in most cases the amount of improvement is more modest and more gradual.

How Your Visual System Works

We created the Power Vision Program for busy people who want hard facts and fast results. This section contains a lot of hard facts and new concepts and may seem complicated, but patiently make your way through it and you'll get a better understanding of how amazing your visual system really is and how it works. You are about to embark on a fascinating journey through the inner workings of the visual system. . . .

We advise you to read this section three times. Even if you don't understand everything at first, don't panic or get frustrated! Persevere and things will soon fall into place. Your eyes are a vitally important part of your life, so learn as much about them as you can! Now for some hard facts.

The eye is an approximately spherical bag of cells about an inch in diameter that is filled with transparent gel and a pressured liquid. At the front is the cornea, which is a transparent window of cells. Behind the cornea is the iris, which is a diaphragm of colored muscle that regulates the amount of light entering the eye.

The pupil is the black hole at the center of the iris through which light passes on its way to the retina. It was recently discovered that the iris is directly connected to breathing! When you inhale, the pupil slightly contracts. When you exhale, it slightly expands.

Behind the iris is the inner lens, which is a flexible capsule of transparent cells with the consistency of rubber. The ciliary muscle surrounds the inner lens and is responsible for focusing it.

The eye's optical system consists of two major components, the cornea and the inner lens. The cornea has almost twice as much focusing power as the inner lens. Light first passes through the cornea, which partially focuses it, then through the inner lens, which completes the process.

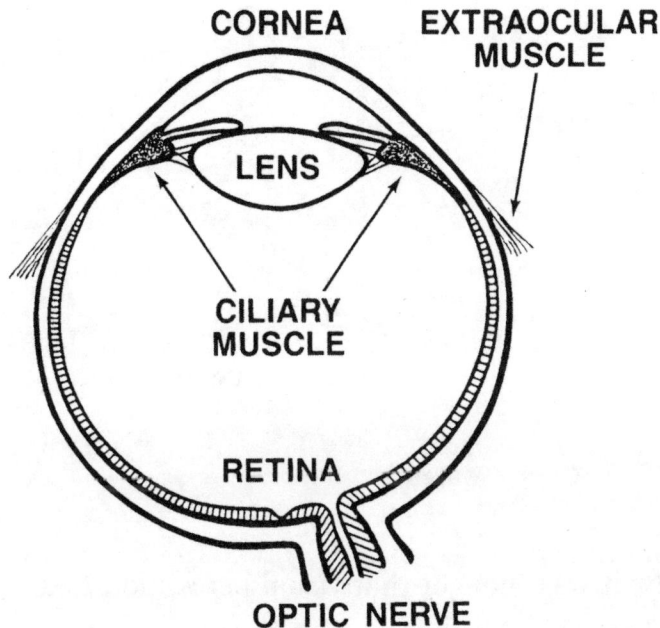

CORNEA   EXTRAOCULAR MUSCLE

LENS

CILIARY MUSCLE

RETINA

OPTIC NERVE

The Zonule of Zinn

The eye changes focus between objects at different distances by the action of the ciliary muscle on the inner lens, which adjusts its shape and refractive power. The ciliary muscle is a circular muscle similar to the iris, and is attached to the inner lens through a meshwork of fibrous filaments known as the *Zonule of Zinn*.

When the ciliary muscle dilates, the zonule pulls on the inner lens and makes it thinner so that it can focus on distant objects. When the ciliary muscle constricts, it presses on the inner lens and makes it thicker by means of what is known as *hydrostatic pressure modulation* of the zonule, so that it can focus on near objects.

As light is focused onto the retina, the rays cross over. This causes the retinal image to be upside down and reversed from left to right. In addition, as a result of optical defects known as *spherical and chromatic aberrations* and *scattering and diffraction*, the retinal image is never perfectly clear, even in perfectly normal eyes.

The retina converts the light into electrical pulses that travel up the optic nerve to the brain, where the image is enhanced by the visual cortex in a process known as *hyperacuity*. It may surprise you to know that what we actually see is 10 times clearer than the raw image on the retina!

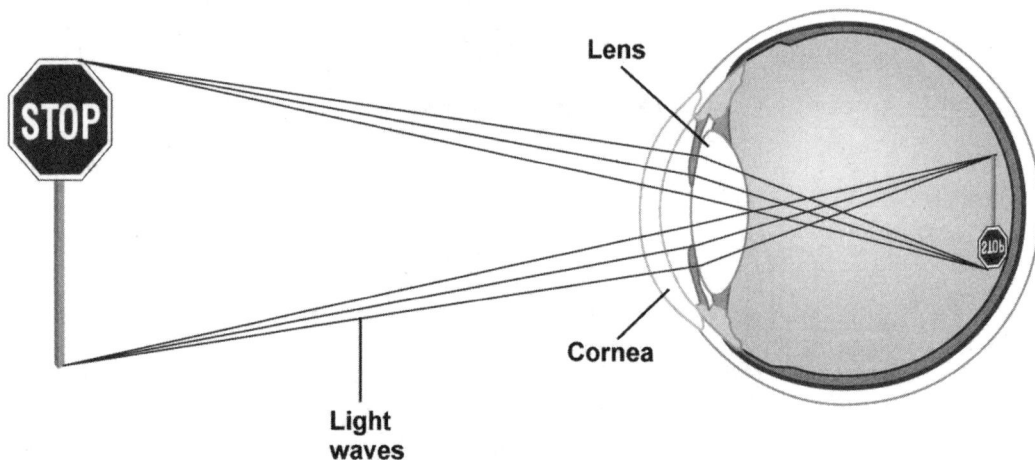

Until recently, it was thought that visual perception takes place in the brain. It is now known that the retina, which is a highly organized network of nerve cells, processes the raw image for basic information such as outlines, colors, and motion. In fact, the retina possesses a rudimentary form of intelligence, and many scientists regard it as an extension of the brain.

The visual cortex then completes the processing and derives more information about detail, distance, and dimension. It adds meaning and integrates the data into what you actually see.

Vision Is Teamwork

Six extraocular muscles surround each eyeball and move the eyes so that they point at the same object at the same time. Their power and precision is truly amazing. It takes about one-tenth of a second for the eyes to jump from one object to another. These rapid eye movements are called *saccades*.

During a saccade, the eyes accelerate at an enormous rate and decelerate almost instantly. To generate enough power, the extraocular muscles are about 200 times stronger than would be needed to slowly turn the eyes in their sockets!

Your eyes are constantly looking from object to object as they scan the world and gather information. For example, as you read these words, your eyes are jumping from one group of letters to the next through a series of saccades.

When you follow a moving object, your eyes make a different type of movement called a *pursuit*. Finally, there is another type of eye movement known as *slow drifting*. If you gaze at an object for more than a few seconds, the eyes will drift away, then return to the object.

In normal, healthy eyes, the ciliary and extraocular muscles work together as a team, constantly adjusting to the world around us. The brain is in complete control and makes the eyes point and focus on the same object at the same time as it constantly searches for objects of interest.

If the teamwork breaks down, the eyes can go out of focus or each eye may point at a different object. This is usually experienced as blurred vision, double vision, eyestrain, slow reading, headaches, poor depth perception, or a tendency to bump into things.

Finally, because the eyes are a few inches apart, each eye receives a slightly different image, which the brain fuses together to form a three-dimensional representation of the world. By improving the coordination of the ciliary and extraocular muscles, vision therapy eye exercises can make the world more real, vivid, and meaningful.

Learn to See for Yourself

Although major advances were made in understanding the eye's anatomy and mode of operation in the nineteenth century, it was discovered in the 1930s that vision is learned. This came as a big surprise because it was previously assumed that vision is automatic.

Although we are born with basic visual reflexes, we learn how to use our eyes. In fact, vision consists of more than a dozen different functions that are learned during childhood through basic experiences.

In addition to forming images, vision gives us the ability to determine the size, speed, distance, and position of an object; the ability to estimate its weight, texture, composition, and age without touching it; the ability to maintain one's sense of balance, posture, and direction; and the ability to read and interpret written words, signs, and symbols.

Like any other learned ability, vision can be improved by practice. This vitally important fact forms the foundation of vision therapy eye exercises. You should not limit yourself by thinking that you are too old or your vision is too bad. The visual system is surprisingly flexible, and older people often get better results than younger people.

Developmental Visual Problems

Like most people, you probably believe that 20/20 is perfect vision. This is an old point of view dating back to the time when the eye care profession was in its infancy. Nowadays, behavioral optometrists realize that what are known as *developmental visual problems* can have a major negative impact on a person's life without the person even realizing it.

Because vision is learned, the amount of learning and hence the development of the visual system depends on the person's experiences. For example, children raised in bright, colorful homes with lots of visual stimuli usually have better visual systems than children raised in dingy squalor. The result is better reading, better comprehension, and higher scores on intelligence tests.

When a child mispronounces a word, the parent notices the error and corrects it. In this way, the child receives feedback and learns how to speak correctly. However, when children learn how to use their eyes, it's impossible for parents to know if the process is proceeding smoothly, unless there are obvious defects such as a lazy eye or crossed eyes.

Many children have 20/20 acuity but are burdened by hidden developmental visual problems. Unless these problems are discovered and corrected, they usually continue unnoticed throughout the person's entire lifetime, causing endless frustration, failure, and underachievement.

For example, people with poor saccadic eye movements usually have difficulty reading or adding up numbers, and are less likely to succeed at school and in the workplace.

Likewise, people with a lazy eye or poor peripheral vision are more likely to bump into things and have accidents.

Developmental visual problems can be superimposed on other visual problems such as myopia, astigmatism, or presbyopia. A behavioral optometrist will detect any developmental visual problems that may be present and prescribe the appropriate course of treatment.

In many cases the result is faster reading with fewer errors, better comprehension, and higher self-esteem. Intellect may also blossom. In one case, the person's IQ score increased by 15 points after vision therapy, simply because the brain was no longer burdened by an inefficient visual system!

Vision Is a Six-Step Process

Basic vision is an amazing six-step process that usually takes less than a second from start to finish.

Step 1: The brain observes the world using peripheral vision, then sees an object of interest and decides to gather information about it. At this stage, the eyes are not pointing directly at the object.

Step 2: The brain then determines the relative position of the object and computes the trajectory and power needed to move the eyes to point directly at it.

Step 3: The brain then directs the extraocular muscles to move the eyes so that they point directly at the object.

Step 4: The brain then directs the ciliary muscle of each eye to focus its lens to make the object clearer.

Step 5: The brain then generates a three-dimensional image of the object, gathers information about it, and determines its significance.

Step 6: Finally, the brain decides whether or not to respond to the object and uses the eyes to coordinate whatever bodily movements are needed.

Clearly, there's a lot more to good vision then meets the eye. . . .

Windows of the Soul

With their enchanting beauty and sex appeal, the eyes are like a delicate exotic flower reaching for the light. Much of this beauty comes from the iris, which has the shape of a colorful wheel with radiant spokes. Quick to protect the retina from potentially harmful glare, the iris can shrink the center of the wheel—the pupil—to the size of a pinhead. In the dark, the iris can expand the pupil up to one-third of an inch to welcome any available light.

Although the iris automatically responds to light, it is also a sensitive barometer of emotion. Anger, fear, pleasure, and lust can be read in the movement of the iris and the size of the pupil. Negative emotions make the iris contract as if to shut out the offending object. Likewise, an expanding pupil registers hidden attraction, as the eye opens up to feast on light from the object of desire.

Eyelids enhance the beauty of the eyes but have a more important function. By blinking every few seconds, they bathe and polish the cornea with antiseptic tears, which protect it against dryness, pollution, bacteria, and foreign objects. Intense emotions can also bring about this purge, and the brain can use tear fluid to eliminate stress-related toxins.

Intense nearpoint work such as long periods of reading or working at a computer can seriously impact tear formation, leading to dry, aching, itching eyes. One of the main goals of the Power Vision Program is to improve tear fluid production and help you avoid these harmful, unpleasant symptoms.

Mirror of the Mind

Quick to capture the beauty of the world, the eyes are also a mirror of the mind. Not only does the iris betray hidden feelings, but the brain uses the eyelids, eyebrows, and eye movements as a subtle means of communication. Because of their remarkable versatility, Saint Jerome wrote, "Eyes without speaking confess the secrets of the heart."

Our language is replete with expressions such as "blind with rage," or "starry eyed," or "his eyes narrowed as he reached for his gun," or "she flashed her eyes at him," or "she gave him the evil eye." Eye contact is an important part of body language. Good eye contact is essential to bonding, whereas a refusal to look someone in the eye is usually a sign of fear or guilt.

When you say "I see," you usually mean more than just looking. You mean "I understand." Throughout the ages, the words *vision, comprehension, intelligence,* and *insight* have interwoven and overlapped in their meaning. This is not an accident of language. It is because vision and intelligence are so closely connected in the human brain.

Vision dominates your life because it is the major link between your brain and the outside world. It is the great channel of communication through which you learn about the world and, ultimately, about yourself.

The Power Vision Program will enhance the beauty and attractiveness of your eyes. Palming and hydrotherapy will literally make your eyes sparkle with new health and vitality, and many people report that the exercises reduce wrinkles, leading to a happier, more youthful appearance!

Your Vision Is Unique

You probably think that everybody sees pretty much the same. Wrong. In fact, people see things differently. Just as each person has a different way of walking, talking, and clothing themselves, each person's visual system is different.

Approximately 5% of people see the world as completely flat! These are usually people with a lazy eye or crossed eyes, who cannot combine the separate images from each eye into three dimensions. About 5% of people have defective color vision, and about 3% of people have developmental visual problems.

Improving your vision can be a profound learning experience, a fascinating period of personal growth and development that will fill you with a sense of pride and accomplishment. As you enhance your visual system, you'll become a happier, more positive person with healthier, more attractive eyes!

Now for Some Basic Terms

Accommodation. The ability to change focus between near and far.

Acuity. Clarity of vision, usually expressed as a fraction such as 20/50. The smaller the denominator, the better the acuity. Far acuity is usually measured at 20 feet and near acuity at 14 inches. Normal vision is defined as 20/20 far acuity or 14/14 near acuity.

Amblyopia (lazy eye). A visual problem in which the brain suppresses nerve impulses from one eye, often leading to subnormal acuity and inferior vision in that eye, and the inability to see the world in three dimensions.

Astigmatism. A visual problem in which the eyeball and/or cornea is warped. The result is uneven focusing of light on the retina so that the image is blurred or distorted, usually at all distances. Astigmatism often occurs in combination with myopia or presbyopia.

Cataracts. A degenerative disease caused by dead cells inside the eye's inner lens, which make the lens cloudy and obstruct the passage of light. A cataract is not a tumor but is usually caused by ultraviolet radiation or poor nutrition. Inner lenses with cataracts can be removed surgically and replaced with artificial inner lenses, but complications from surgery sometimes cause blindness.

Ciliary muscle. The circular muscle that surrounds the inner lens and makes it change shape.

Convergence. The ability to point the eye at the same object at the same time.

Corrective lenses. Glasses or contacts that treat blurred vision by compensating for the eye's optical defects. They don't correct the underlying problem but merely bend the light before it enters the eye. Corrective lenses are also known as *compensatory lenses*.

Developmental problems. Visual problems that arise when a child's visual system fails to develop properly. A child may have 20/20 acuity but have problems with convergence or accommodation. Developmental problems can remain undetected throughout the person's entire lifetime.

Diopter. The unit of measurement of the strength of a lens. The stronger the lens, the more diopters it has.

Dry eye disease. A condition in which the tear glands don't produce enough tear fluid or produce tear fluid with the wrong composition.

Environmental theory. The theory that environmental factors such as stress, lighting, nutrition, posture, and too much close work are the major cause of common visual problems such as eyestrain, astigmatism, and myopia.

Genetic theory. The theory that visual problems are inherited or genetically determined.

Glaucoma. A degenerative disease in which the optic nerve is damaged due to poor blood supply and/or excess pressure inside the eyeball, usually caused by blockages in the eye's drainage system. Glaucoma can lead to total blindness.

Hyperopia (farsightedness). A visual problem in which far objects are seen better than near objects. A farsighted person is called a *hyperope* (pronounced *HYPER-ope*).

Laser surgery. The use of a laser to destroy cellular tissue. Lasers are used to treat glaucoma by drilling tiny drainage holes to relieve the pressure. Lasers are also used to treat myopia and astigmatism by vaporizing part of the cornea, thereby changing its curvature and refractive power.

Macular degeneration. A degenerative disease in which cells die in the central part of the retina at the back of the eye, usually resulting in partial blindness.

Minus lenses. Lenses that make objects appear smaller. Minus lenses have negative refractive power such as −5.00D and are used to treat the symptoms of myopia.

Myopia (nearsightedness). A visual problem in which the person sees near objects better than far objects. A nearsighted person is called a *myope* (pronounced *MY-ope*). Myopia is often accompanied by astigmatism.

Myopia morbidity. Degenerative diseases caused by or associated with myopia, including cataracts, glaucoma, and retinal detachment. Myopia is officially listed as a major cause of blindness.

Nearpoint stress. The major visual stress factor caused by doing too much reading; spending too much time looking at computers, TV, or smartphones; or staring at close objects for extended periods of time.

Ophthalmologist. An eye doctor who treats eye diseases with drugs and/or surgery. Many ophthalmologists also prescribe corrective lenses or perform refractive surgery such as LASIK.

Optician. A technician who dispenses glasses and contact lenses.

Optometrist. A traditional optometrist is an eye doctor who treats visual problems with corrective lenses. A behavioral optometrist treats visual problems with vision therapy eye exercises and corrective lenses if necessary. Optometrists also prescribe drugs and perform minor surgery.

Peripheral vision. The ability to see out of the corner of your eyes, enabling you to detect shapes without looking directly at them. It's essential for recognizing potential threats, avoiding obstacles, and maintaining spatial orientation.

Plus lenses. Lenses that make objects appear bigger. Plus lenses have positive refractive power such as +2.00D.

Presbyopia (aging eyes). Loss of focusing power due to the aging process. A person with presbyopia is called a *presbyope* (pronounced *PREZ-bee-ope*). Presbyopia occurs in addition to existing visual problems such as myopia or astigmatism.

Progressive undercorrection. The use of a series of weaker corrective lenses in conjunction with vision therapy eye exercises to reduce the eye's refractive error.

Refractive power. A measurement in diopters of the eye's inability to focus light onto the retina.

Strabismus (crossed eyes). A visual problem where the eyes point in different directions, causing double vision or suppressed vision in one eye.

Therapeutic lenses. Lenses that improve visual performance and enhance comfort, including lenses to reduce refractive error and remediate developmental problems such as strabismus.

Vision therapy. Techniques that improve the performance of the visual system, including acupressure, behavior modification, biofeedback, hydrotherapy, hypnosis, nutrition, ocular calisthenics, stress reduction, syntonics, yoga, and therapeutic lenses.

What Really Causes Bad Eyesight

Traditional eye care is based on the unproven theory that common visual problems such as myopia, hyperopia, and astigmatism are the result of genetically deformed eyeballs, which are either too long, or too short, or warped.

The truth is that humans evolved to have excellent eyesight, especially at a distance, because our ancestors were hunters and warriors whose survival depended on it. People with bad eyesight were killed by enemies and predators, so they didn't survive. The fact that humans survived and thrived is proof that we are genetically programmed for excellent eyesight.

The problem is that mass education, TV, smartphones, computers, and spending long periods of time indoors force many people to look at close objects for hour after hour. This causes the ciliary muscles and extraocular muscles to malfunction. Blinking and tear formation are also reduced. The result is known as *nearpoint stress*. This increases the pressure inside the eyeball, which can gradually elongate it.

But you may ask, "My parents are myopic and I am also myopic. Doesn't that mean the myopia is inherited?" The answer is, "No!" The reason why myopia often seems to be inherited is because parents and children share a similar lifestyle, such as watching a lot of TV, or doing a lot of reading or computer work, or playing a lot of video games.

Professor Young, coauthor of the Power Vision Program, explains:

"Just because parents and children speak the same language doesn't mean that language is inherited. It simply means that parents and children are exposed to the same culture. The same thing applies to myopia."

The aging process is another major cause of bad eyesight. The lens loses its flexibility and the ciliary muscles lose their focusing power, so that near objects must be held farther away. The circulation of nutrients in and around the eyes also declines, increasing the risk of cataracts, glaucoma, and macular degeneration.

The traditional method of treating visual problems is with corrective lenses—which don't really correct anything. If they did, you'd wear them for a while, and then you wouldn't need them anymore because your visual problem would have been corrected.

All they do is treat the symptoms, the blur, by bending light before it enters the eyes. But they don't correct the visual problem itself, which is usually nearpoint stress, or malfunction of the ciliary muscle, or the aging process. To avoid misleading their patients, behavioral optometrists usually refer to corrective lenses as *compensatory lenses*. In fact, no clinical studies have proved the long-term safety or effectiveness of corrective lenses.

What Corrective Lenses Do to Your Eyes

Now for some hard facts about the optical glass industry.

The invention of lenses about 800 years ago is one of the major accomplishments of Western civilization. In addition to helping millions of people see more clearly, lenses are an integral part of important scientific instruments such as microscopes and telescopes, which have opened our eyes to the hidden wonders of the world and deepened our understanding of the universe. It is no exaggeration to say that the optical glass industry has made and continues to make a major contribution to our modern way of life.

The big problem with corrective lenses is the traditional way of prescribing them, which treats the symptoms but ignores the underlying visual problem. As you probably know from your own experience, corrective lenses usually create dependency and make the eyes weaker. After a year or two, a stronger prescription is needed, which increases dependency and makes the eyes even weaker.

The result is a vicious cycle of dependency and deterioration, causing a gradual loss of vision, with progressively stronger corrective lenses making the eyes progressively weaker. In many cases, this leads to a degenerative disease such as cataracts, glaucoma, or retinal detachment.

In a series of important experiments, Dr. Earl Smith of the University of Houston College of Optometry fitted corrective lenses on monkeys with *normal* vision. What he discovered shocked the eye care establishment.

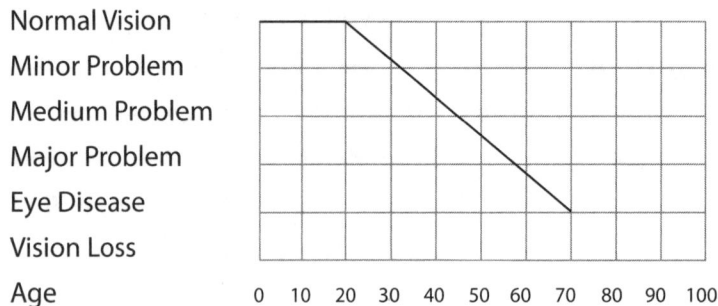

Normal Vision	
Minor Problem	
Medium Problem	
Major Problem	
Eye Disease	
Vision Loss	
Age	0 10 20 30 40 50 60 70 80 90 100

Monkeys fitted with corrective lenses for myopia adapted to the lenses and became myopic! Same thing happened to monkeys fitted with corrective lenses for astigmatism. They adapted to the lenses and developed astigmatism! Same thing with corrective lenses for farsightedness.

The implications of this research are of serious concern because the visual systems of monkeys and humans are almost identical. Simply stated, the evidence shows that corrective lenses can cause or aggravate common visual problems.

In fact, the traditional way of prescribing corrective lenses can turn a minor focusing error into a serious visual problem. Our research and that of other scientists and behavioral optometrists leaves no doubt that corrective lenses can cause the eyes to lose even more of their natural focusing ability, and that reading through corrective lenses is the major cause of progressive myopia.

Professor Young explains:

Monkeys fitted with corrective lenses for myopia adapted to the lenses and became myopic! Same thing happened to monkeys fitted with corrective lenses for astigmatism.

"The worst thing you can do for myopia is to treat it with corrective lenses. These increase the level of accommodation when worn for close work and cause further deterioration. If treated with vision therapy and therapeutic lenses, myopia should be a transitory condition like a headache that goes away. Instead, corrective lenses aggravate the problem and condemn the patient to a lifetime of dependency."

Concerned Doctors Speak Out

Over the years, many other doctors have also voiced their concerns:

"Full correction for distance vision causes the myope to produce extra accommodation when viewing close objects with their lenses on. This can cause the eye to become more myopic when fully corrected."

J. Angle & D. A. Wissman, *Soc. Sci. Med.*, 14A: 473–479, 1980

"Minus lenses for full-time use produce accommodative insufficiency associated with additional symptoms until the patient gets used to the lenses. This is usually accompanied by a further increase in myopia and the cycle begins anew."

M. H. Birnbaum, *Rev. Optom.*, 110(21): 23–29, 1973

"The emphasis on compensatory lenses has posed a problem for many years in our examinations. These lenses do not correct anything and may not serve the patient in his best interests over a period of time."

C. J. Forkiotis, *OEP*, 53:1, 1980

"Spectacle lenses can create their own problems. There are frequently ignored patterns of addiction to minus lenses. The typical prescription tends to overpower and fatigue the visual system and what should be a transient condition becomes a lifelong situation, which is likely to deteriorate over time."

S. Gallop, *J. Behav. Optom.*, 5(5): 115–120, 1994

"The use of compensatory lenses to treat or neutralize the symptoms does not correct or cure the problem. The current education and training of eye care professionals discourages preventive and remedial treatment."

R. L. Gottlieb, *J. Optom. Vis. Dev.*, 13(1): 3–27, 1982

"I'm sure that most optometrists will confirm the clinical observation that patients who receive compensatory lenses for full-time wear are usually the ones who need a stronger prescription every year."

J. Liberman, *J. Am. Optom. Assoc.*, 47(8): 1058–1064, 1976

"Concave lenses are the most common approach, yet the least likely to prevent myopic progression. Unfortunately, they increase the nearpoint stress that is associated with progression."

B. May, *OEP*, A(1120), 1984

Understanding Eye Doctors

Optometrists and ophthalmologists are highly skilled health care professionals who are trained to practice what is known as *traditional eye care*. This consists of checking for disease, prescribing drugs and corrective lenses, and performing eye surgery. However, the vast majority of patients who rely on corrective lenses become progressively worse.

To give credit where credit is due, the optical glass industry produces high-quality products at easily affordable prices, and corrective lenses have helped millions of people live happier and more productive lives. These products provide a *quick fix*—which most people are satisfied with and benefit from, at least in the short term.

Our concern is that corrective lenses are a major risk factor for cataracts, glaucoma, and macular degeneration. The reason is that corrective lenses, especially bifocals, interfere with the activity of the ciliary muscle and inner lens. This affects the fluid dynamics and the flow of nutrients inside the eye and the expulsion of cellular waste products, making it more prone to degenerative diseases.

Fortunately, a significant number of eye care professionals have advanced beyond the traditional use of corrective lenses. Behavioral optometrists treat the underlying cause of visual problems—not just the symptoms—and their patients usually get better, not worse. Of course, they will prescribe corrective lenses for patients who just want a quick fix.

Although corrective lenses will continue to play an important role for people who just want a quick fix, much more can be done. Good vision care means exercising your eyes, just like good physical health means exercising your body. It makes a lot of sense, and it works!

The Emperor Has No Clothes

Although more than 150,000 research papers have been published on the eyes, some vitally important topics have never been investigated. These topics involve the long-term effects of corrective lenses on the ciliary muscle, extraocular muscles, and inner lens.

Merely to say that there are large gaps in our knowledge is an understatement. In fact, almost nothing is known about the long-term effects of corrective lenses on the visual system except that the vast majority of people who rely on them become progressively worse and require stronger prescriptions every few years. In some cases, every few months!

Simply stated, no clinical studies have demonstrated the long-term safety or effectiveness of corrective lenses. Likewise, not a single clinical study has ever been published showing that the traditional use of corrective lenses has cured or even improved any of the common visual problems! In other words, if you are wearing corrective lenses, you are using what is basically an untested and unproven method of treatment.

For this reason, we advise you to use glasses as tools for specific tasks and remove them when the task is complete. Of course, you must always wear glasses that enable you to see well for potentially dangerous activities such as driving, crossing the road, and using power tools or kitchen utensils.

It's not difficult to understand why research has not been carried out in this area. The optical glass industry generates billions of dollars every year from corrective lenses—as do the doctors who prescribe them. Most patients are happy with the quick fix that corrective lenses give them, so there's no incentive for the eye care establishment to carry out research into the long-term effects of these products.

Our concern is that despite the modern advances in vision care, the eye care establishment uses the same old method of prescribing corrective lenses that was developed hundreds of years ago—and the vast majority of their patients get worse!

However, there's another reason why most traditional eye care professionals don't take advantage of advances in vision care. Almost all ophthalmologists only read journals dealing with ophthalmology. Likewise, almost all traditional optometrists only read journals dealing with traditional optometry.

Many advances in vision research are published in journals dealing with psychology, ergonomics, behavioral optometry, and other areas of investigation. Traditional optometrists and ophthalmologists don't read these journals and aren't aware of these advances. For this reason, it can take decades for research discoveries to make their way into the courses that are taught in traditional optometric colleges and medical schools.

How the Eyes Adapt

As a result of decades of research and clinical observations, we have concluded that the eyes adapt to corrective lenses by gradually changing their form and function. Professor Allen, coauthor of the Power Vision Program, explains:

> "Whenever a lens is placed in front of the eye, the eye will gradually adapt its form and function in order to minimize the energy required to focus the inner lens. The situation is like wearing a finger ring. After wearing the ring for a few months, the finger adapts by forming a slight groove beneath the ring."

Clearly, there's something really wrong with the traditional method of treatment. As a general principle in health care, patients should get better, not worse. With traditional eye care, however, once a patient starts wearing corrective lenses, it's usually downhill all the way—often ending up with a potentially blinding disease such as cataract or retinal detachment.

Even worse, one of the most harmful myths perpetrated by the eye care establishment is that going without corrective lenses will damage your eyes. There's not a shred of evidence to support this point of view. On the contrary, going without corrective lenses is one of the most important vision therapy techniques, because it breaks the vicious cycle of dependency and deterioration.

That's why you shouldn't use the Power Vision Program under the care of a traditional optometrist or ophthalmologist, who will probably tell you that they have not seen any evidence that eye exercises work. The reason, as we previously explained, is that they have not read the journals where the evidence is published and are not familiar with the advances that have been made.

Having said that, we must emphasize that the vast majority of traditional eye doctors are not villains! On the contrary, they are decent, hard-working professionals who earn their living and pay off their student loans by doing what they have been trained to do, which is to serve their patients by providing a quick fix.

For best results, we recommend that you do the therapy under the care of a behavioral optometrist. You can get a referral from *www.oepf.org* or *www.covd.org*. If they can't refer you to anyone in your area, look for an optometrist who already offers vision therapy.

Before having an eye exam, leave the Power Vision Program with the optometrist and ask if they are willing to help you. Shop around until you find an optometrist who is enthusiastic about helping you achieve your goals. If you can't afford professional vision care, you can use the Power Vision Program on your own. Read everything three times or until you understand the main points, and make sure you understand the exercises and procedures. Do everything as directed, and don't take shortcuts.

Set Yourself Realistic Goals

The Power Vision Program is designed to make your eyes healthier, increase your natural focusing power, and help you avoid corrective lenses or reduce your dependency on them. However, this doesn't mean that everybody will regain 20/20 acuity. Based on our clinical experience with more than 1,000 patients, we have determined that the Power Vision Program can usually produce the following improvements:

Group One: If your vision is not too bad and you're wearing your first pair of glasses, or you don't wear them and think you need them, you can probably return to normal and avoid them. It should only take a few weeks to get results.

Group Two: If you've worn glasses for more than a year and your vision is getting worse, you can probably avoid having to get a stronger prescription. The Power Vision Program will help you see well with your current prescription, and it should take only a few weeks to get results.

Group Three: If you've worn glasses for more than a year and want to get the maximum improvement from the Power Vision Program, you can probably reach the point where you can use a weaker prescription and need it only part-time. The rest of the time, you'll be able to see quite well without glasses. It usually takes two or three months to get the maximum improvement. Some people will be able to get rid of them altogether.

Although most people see the first signs of improvement in about a week, don't be impatient or discouraged if you don't get results right away. Be realistic and give the exercises time to work. The important thing is to develop the habit of doing one or more of the exercise modules every day.

Use Corrective Lenses Therapeutically

When people get a new pair of glasses, they usually must get used to the stronger lenses. This usually takes a few weeks as the eyes passively adapt to the stronger lenses.

We have discovered that the same principle can be used in reverse. Instead of passively adapting to stronger lenses, it is possible to actively adapt to a series of weaker lenses using eye exercises to make the eyes stronger and increase their focusing ability.

In this process, which is important for Group Three, weaker glasses are used therapeutically to treat the underlying visual problem, not just the symptoms. The eye exercises increase the range and power of your eye's focusing mechanism and help you adapt to the weaker lenses. When you can see well through the weaker lenses, use even weaker lenses. We call this process *progressive undercorrection*.

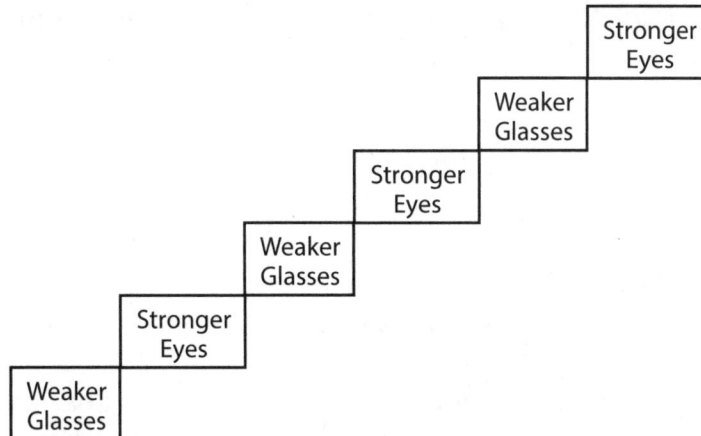

Weaker glasses from previous years can often be used. If you are myopic, the weaker glasses must give you 20/40 acuity so that you can drive safely. If your glasses are already weak, use them until you can see well through them; then use even weaker glasses. If you are hyperopic or presbyopic, you can probably use drugstore glasses. Get the weakest pair you can read with.

If you don't have any weaker glasses, you can get some from a behavioral optometrist or a company such as Lenscrafters, which usually takes a few days. Make sure the optometrist understands that you want a 20/40 undercorrection. When ready, check the glasses and make sure that things are slightly blurred. You only need new lenses, not new frames.

Strategies for Success

We recommend that you get a comprehensive eye exam to make sure there aren't any diseases or developmental problems that require specialized treatment. You should also schedule weekly meetings with your optometrist to review your progress and resolve any issues that may arise.

We also recommend the following general strategies. If you are myopic, don't read or use a computer or do any type of close work through distance glasses, because this will cause more nearpoint stress. However, regardless of your visual problem, you must always wear corrective lenses that enable you to see well when doing any type of potentially dangerous activity.

Group One: Avoid straining your eyes from too much reading or computer work. If you already wear glasses, go without them as much as possible provided it's safe to do so. However, behavioral optometrists often prescribe therapeutic *low plus* lenses to reduce nearpoint stress, which should be worn as directed.

Group Two: Although your goal is to see well with your current glasses, break the habit of leaving them on all the time. Use them as tools that help you accomplish a specific activity, and remove them when you finish the activity.

Group Three: Go without corrective lenses as much as possible provided it's safe to do so. Wear weaker glasses and concentrate on adapting to them. When you can see well through the weaker glasses, go back to even weaker glasses. The weaker glasses should give you 20/40 acuity so that things are slightly blurred but not so blurred that you can't make them out.

How to Use Contact Lenses Effectively

If you're nearsighted and do a lot of reading or computer work, we advise you not to wear contact lenses unless you get special lenses for close work. You will need contact lenses that give you 20/40 acuity at a distance of 20 inches.

If you don't do much reading or computer work, it's okay to wear weaker contact lenses that give you 20/40 acuity for distant objects. We recommend disposable contacts.

The Three Phases of Vision Therapy

The most important thing is to generate momentum and enthusiasm as quickly as possible. Get up to speed and see the results for yourself. That's the key to success. Once you feel the changes taking place in your eyes and see the first signs of improvement, you'll know beyond a shadow of doubt that you made the right decision and are moving in the right direction.

You'll experience such a tremendous feeling of satisfaction and accomplishment that you'll never look back! You'll never want to go back to the traditional method of treatment, where you're trapped in a vicious cycle of weaker eyes and stronger prescriptions.

Phase One: Learning

During the first couple of weeks, your goal is to become familiar with all the exercises so you can do them without referring to the book. Read the instructions carefully and make sure you're doing them correctly. After a few days, you'll be able to do them without referring to the book.

Reduce your dependency on corrective lenses as quickly as possible unless your goal is to avoid a stronger prescription, in which case concentrate on seeing better through your current glasses. Diligently cultivate your new visual habits by doing vision therapy at traffic lights, during TV and YouTube commercial breaks, and when standing in line.

Phase Two: Development

This is a period of rapid progress where your goal is to get the improvement you need to achieve your goals. If your vision is not too bad and you want to avoid glasses, or your vision is bad and you want to avoid a stronger prescription, you can probably do this within a month.

If your vision is bad and you want to maximize the amount of improvement and enjoy freedom from glasses, it usually takes two or three months. During this time, you'll master the exercises and figure out which are working best for you.

Phase Three: Maintenance

In this phase, you'll rely on your new visual habits to maintain the results automatically. You'll be in the habit of spontaneously doing vision therapy at traffic lights, during TV and YouTube commercial breaks, and whenever you are standing in line.

Study Your Blur Zone

Most people have a zone of clear vision and a zone where everything is blurred. If you have a lot of astigmatism, hyperopia, or presbyopia, things may be blurred at all distances. If you have a lot of myopia, your clear zone may extend only a few inches from your eyes.

Nearsighted Person		Clear Zone		Blur Zone

Farsighted Person		Blur Zone		Clear Zone

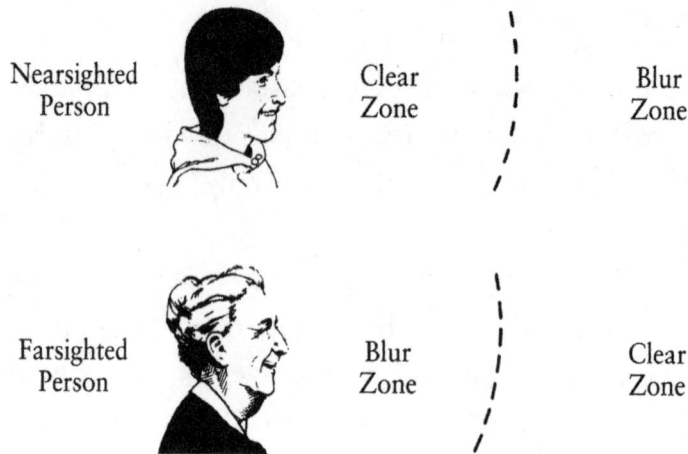

The place where the clear zone ends and the blur zone begins is called the *blur threshold.* By developing the habit of studying blurred objects, especially objects near your blur threshold that are slightly blurred, your clear zone will increase and your acuity will improve.

How to Detect a Lazy Eye

Lazy eye, also known as *amblyopia*, occurs when one eye fails to develop a strong connection to the brain, leading to reduced vision in the affected eye. In extreme cases, it may lead to crossed eyes (strabismus).

Most people have a dominant eye and a weaker eye, like being left-handed or right-handed. The brain does most of its seeing through the dominant eye and uses the weaker eye as confirmation. However, if the weaker eye is abnormally weak, it can lead to problems similar to a lazy eye, such as not seeing in three dimensions or not being able to judge distance. Here's a simple test to help you find out.

Make a large dot on a blank wall and sit about 10 feet in front of it. Now hold the index finger of your dominant hand about 6 inches in front of you and look at the dot. You will see two fingers, one on each side of the dot.

Even if you don't have a lazy eye or an abnormally weak eye, we strongly recommend using an eyepatch to fully develop your eyes and balance your visual system.

The left finger corresponds to the right eye, and vice versa. Notice if one of the fingers is fainter than the other one. If so, the fainter finger corresponds to your weaker eye. If it is much fainter, you probably have an abnormally weak eye or a lazy eye.

The Importance of Patching

The best way to treat a lazy eye or an abnormally weak eye is through patching. If you have either of these problems, you are seeing in only two dimensions without even realizing it. By bringing the weak eye up to par, a new dimension will suddenly appear out of nowhere and you'll experience the world as you've never seen it before!

Even if you don't have a lazy eye or an abnormally weak eye, we strongly recommend using an eyepatch to fully develop your eyes and balance your visual system. As a result, the world will become brighter and you'll see more vividly in three dimensions. Using an eyepatch often produces the *wow effect*, so don't skip it.

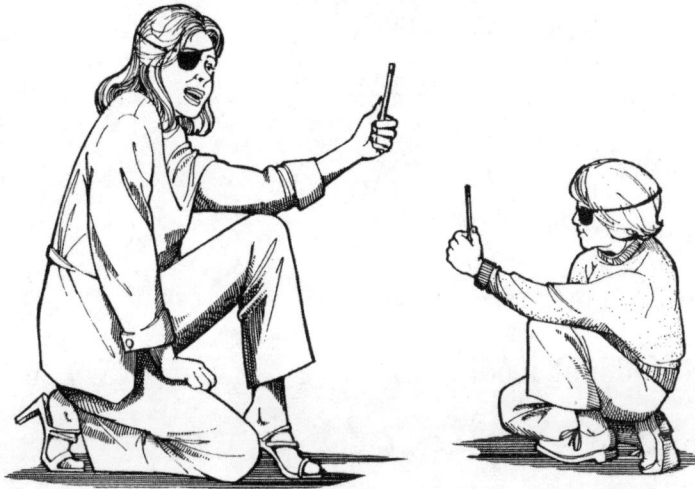

Get an eyepatch from a drugstore, and wear it for about an hour a day when reading, watching television, or playing. Patch each eye in turn. Patch your dominant eye about three times as long as the weaker eye. This will force the brain to use the weaker eye, which will make your visual system more efficient. You should also do extra Flexing, Detailing, and Biofeedback with the eyepatch in place.

Using an eye patch can really accelerate your progress, and we strongly recommend that you get one! Don't wear it for potentially dangerous activities such as driving, crossing the road, or using power tools or kitchen utensiles.

Stress and Nutrition

Vision is the major link between your brain and the world because most of your experiences come through your eyes. Approximately 35% of your brain's cortex is devoted to operating your visual system. For this reason, it's important to reduce all forms of stress, especially nearpoint stress. The best way of reducing nearpoint stress is through Slow Blinking and the Booster module exercises.

You should also optimize your nutrition so your brain has enough fuel to operate your visual system efficiently. We endorse the recommendations of the American Cancer Society and the National Institutes of Health:

- Eat less salt.

- Eat less sugar.

- Drink lots of liquids.

- Eat whole-grain cereals.

- Don't add salt to your food.

- Avoid tobacco and junk food.

- Eat lots of fruits and vegetables.

- Take a multivitamin supplement.

Make a Formal Decision to Succeed

You must sincerely believe that you need to make positive changes in your visual system. This means weighing the pros and cons and making an intelligent choice so that you're convinced you're doing the right thing.

Just as the road to hell is paved with good intentions, it's probably true that in many cases, the road to blindness is paved with corrective lenses! In all probability, traditional eye care is leading you on a downward spiral into progressively stronger prescriptions. Common sense dictates that you should turn things around before it's too late. Your goal should be to get better, not worse.

The next step is to make a formal decision such as a written statement or contract with yourself, or a vow, that nothing will stop you from succeeding. Then make your decision public by telling your friends, relatives, and associates. A public commitment is important because it makes you accountable to other people, who will encourage and motivate you.

If you just make a private decision, you can always find an excuse to wriggle out of it. Although you may experience a few pangs of guilt and remorse, your decision will soon be forgotten and you'll continue to deteriorate as your old visual habits reassert themselves. Don't let that happen!

How to Get Really Fast Results

- **Start the program immediately.** Don't procrastinate. Print extra Reminder Cards and Biofeedback Charts. Put them in prominent locations in your home, office, and car. Print the Progress Report and use it to track your progress. Motivate yourself and get results!

- **Read everything three times.** This is very important. You are learning new words and concepts, so re-read everything until you fully understand it, or at least understand the main points.

- **Exercise your eyes every day.** Do at least one of the exercise modules once a day. It only takes about 10 minutes. If you want faster results, do two or three exercise modules.

- **Don't overdo it.** Your eyes will feel sore at first, like any physical exercise program would cause you to feel. *If you feel sharp pain or your eyes become unpleasantly sore, you must immediately stop!* Then do the Booster exercises for a few days or until the discomfort subsides.

- **Rearrange your schedule.** Never resort to the pitiful old excuse that you don't have enough time. Make time! Your eyes are vastly more important than watching TV or talking on the phone. Set aside a special time to do the therapy without being disturbed or distracted. Switch off the TV and put your phone in another room.

- **Do an exercise session in the morning.** That way it's done and you won't get sidetracked and forget. If possible, do another exercise session in the evening.

- **Use an alarm clock.** Habits thrive on regularity, so use an alarm clock to remind yourself. This is the best way of cultivating your positive new habit of doing vision therapy on a regular basis. Using an alarm clock is really important, so don't skip it.

- **Use the Progress Report.** Record your progress every day. Aim for a perfect week where you do an exercise session every day!

- **Don't be lazy.** Don't let laziness or negative thoughts such as "I can't be bothered to exercise today" or "This isn't going to work" sabotage your progress. Do the exercises even if you don't feel like doing them, because they'll lift your mood and make you feel better.

- **Reward yourself.** After doing your daily exercise session, eat some chocolate or fruit or beef jerky or listen to your favorite music. If you have a perfect week, celebrate by giving yourself a big reward. Go shopping and buy something special or have a nice meal at a fancy restaurant.

- **Develop new visual habits.** Resolutely integrate vision therapy with traffic lights, TV and YouTube commercials, and standing in line. Do this until exercising your eyes is part of your normal lifestyle and you don't have to think about it.

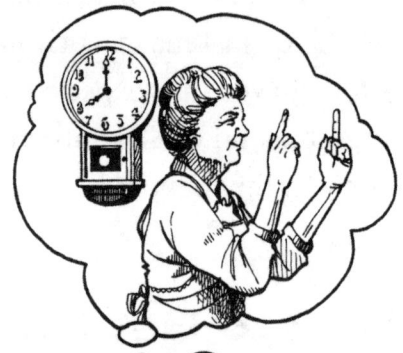

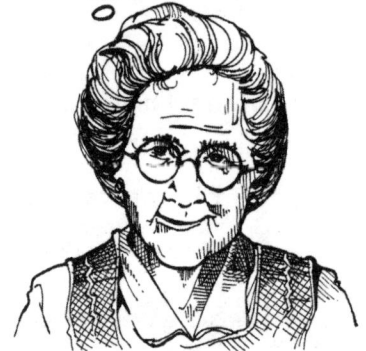

- **Improve your posture.** Bad posture can be a major factor in astigmatism and myopia, and improving it usually results in an improvement in vision.

- **Don't squint or use trick vision.** When doing the exercises and during the course of the day, keep your eyes open and relaxed and accept what you can see for what it is. Don't try to force yourself to see clearly.

- **Wear weaker glasses.** This applies only to Group Three. If you continue to wear your current glasses, you won't get results. However, if your current glasses are already weak, wear them until you can see well with them; then use even weaker glasses.

- **Don't read through distance glasses.** This only applies if you are nearsighted because reading through distance glasses creates nearpoint stress and causes deterioration. Remove your distance glasses for all reading and computer work, even if it means being closer than usual. If you are very myopic, get weaker glasses or contacts that give you 20/40 acuity at 20 inches.

- **Spend time without glasses.** Break the habit of leaving your glasses on all the time. Regard them as tools that you use for activities where you must have good vision, and cultivate the habit of taking them off as soon as you finish the activity.

- **Use the Clearing Sequence.** When looking at a blurred object, develop the habit of doing a Squeeze Blink followed by a few Fast Blinks; then look at the smallest detail you can see, or run your gaze along the edges of the object. This is known as the *Clearing Sequence* because it can improve acuity by forming a natural contact lens composed of tear fluid. Practice it until it becomes part of your normal way of seeing.

- **Wear sunglasses outdoors.** It's important to stop ultraviolet light from entering your eyes because it's a major cause of cataracts and macular degeneration. Get the lightest tint available so that your pupils don't dilate, and make sure the tag states that the sunglasses block ultraviolet light.

- **Use an eyepatch.** Get one from your local drugstore and wear it for one hour a day when reading, watching TV, or playing video games. Patch each eye in turn. If you have an abnormally weak eye or a lazy eye, patch the stronger eye about three times as long as the weak or lazy eye.

- **Use the Potentiation Effect.** When you've mastered the exercises, do some of them for longer periods of time. This gives more improvement than several shorter periods and is known as the *Potentiation Effect*. For example, do 10 minutes of Flexing or 15 minutes of Palming.

- **Upgrade your nutrition.** Avoid food containing sugar, especially carbonated drinks, because sugar can make the inner lens swell up and aggravate myopia. Poor nutrition can also increase the risk of cataracts and macular degeneration. Eat less fat. Drink plenty of water. Eat whole grain cereals. Eat plenty of fruits and vegetables. Don't add salt to your food. Take a good multivitamin supplement.

- **Tell your friends.** If you tell your friends and associates that you're improving your vision with eye exercises, they will follow your progress and encourage you. This will motivate you and keep you on track.

- **Verbally motivate yourself.** Resolutely repeat the affirmation to activate your body's natural healing process: "My eyes are getting better and my vision is improving!" Use the affirmation to neutralize negative thoughts such as "I can't be bothered to do the eye exercises today" or "This isn't going to work." Make copies of the Affirmation Chart and put them at strategic locations such as your bathroom mirror, refrigerator door, or car dashboard. Use the Affirmation Chart as an extra Biofeedback Chart. Repeat the affirmation until it becomes deeply embedded in your subconscious mind!

Affirmation Chart

My Eyes Are Getting Better And My Vision Is Improving! My Eyes Ar e Getting Better And My Vision Is Improving! My Eyes Are Getting Better And My Vision Is Improving! My Eyes Are Getting Better And My Vision Is Improving! My Eyes Are Getting Better And My Vision Is Improving! My Eyes Are Getting Better And My Vision Is Improving! My Eyes Are Getting Better And My Vision Is Improving! My Eyes Are Getting Better And My Vision Is Improving! My Eyes Are Getting Better And My Vision I s Improving! My Eyes Are Getting Better And My Vision Is Improving! My Eyes Are Getting Better And My Vision Is Improving! My Eyes Are Getting Better And My Vision Is Improving! My Eyes Are Getting Better And My Vision Is Improving! My Eyes Are Getting Better And My Vision Is Improving! My Eyes Are Getting Better And My Vision Is Improving! My Eyes Are Getting Better And My Vision Is Improving! My Eyes Are Getting Better And My Vision Is Improving! My Eyes Are Getting Better And My Vision Is Improving! ! My Eye Are Getting Better And My Vision Is Improving! My Eyes Are Getting Better And My Vision Is Improving! My Eyes Are Getting Better And My Vision Is Improving! ! My Eyes Are Getting Better And My Vision Is Improving! My Eyes Are Getting Better And My Vision Is Improving! My Eyes Are Getting

Signs of Progress

During the first week, pay special attention to how your eyes feel, and keep reminding yourself to do the therapy. Soon you'll notice the first signs of habit formation. Perhaps you'll be at a traffic light, or channel hopping, or standing in line at a grocery store and your mind will be a million miles away, dreaming of something else.

Suddenly, without thinking about it, you'll spontaneously do some Squeeze Blinking, or Fast Blinking, or Detailing. You'll experience a burst of excitement as you realize your new visual habits are taking root in your subconscious mind. As the days go by, you'll find yourself spontaneously practicing your new visual habits more and more often.

As the therapy takes effect, interesting and often dramatic improvements may take place. If you are myopic, your blur zone will start to move away from you and distant objects will become clearer. If you are hyperopic or presbyopic, the opposite will occur. If you have astigmatism, objects at all distances will start to become clearer.

If you're wearing a weaker prescription, you'll start to see more clearly through it. If you just want to stabilize your vision, you'll start to see more clearly through your current prescription. You may also experience *clear flashes* where everything is perfectly clear. These can take place with a weaker prescription or during your time without glasses.

You'll also develop a more vivid awareness of the world, which will appear to be more solid and three-dimensional. Colors will become brighter, and your eyes will feel as if they are more open and alive. You'll also become more confident and relaxed with a sense of power and control, knowing that you're accomplishing something important for your future and your well-being.

Positive changes will also occur in the form and function of your eyes. These changes are inevitable because eye exercises increase the flow of nutrients to the eyes and improve the operation of the eye muscles. These factors must produce positive changes at a cellular level. The laws of nature must be obeyed!

If you ever feel tempted to quit, remember this: The vast majority of people who rely on corrective lenses get worse. They are on a downward spiral of progressively stronger lenses, often ending up with a serious eye disease such as cataracts or retinal detachment. Don't follow that route! Vision therapy eye exercises have worked for thousands of people like yourself. They will work for you too.

Master all the exercises. Depending on your visual problem, you'll find that some exercises are more effective than others or that you gravitate to some of the exercises and enjoy doing them. Concentrate on those exercises and incorporate them into your lifestyle so they become part of your normal way of seeing.

Putting It All Together

Improving your vision is easy if you follow these steps:

- Do at least one exercise module every day.

- Practice your new visual habits at traffic lights, during TV and YouTube commercial breaks, and when standing in line.

- Use glasses as tools to help you accomplish specific tasks and remove them when you finish the task. Break the habit of leaving them on all the time.

The only problem you're likely to encounter is motivation. Basically, your task is to replace your negative old habits with positive new ones. If possible, do the exercises with a friend or coworker so you motivate and encourage each other.

It will take about a month to firmly establish your positive new habits. During this period, you'll probably experience resistance from your old habits and subconscious mind in the form of a bad attitude or negative thoughts and emotions, such as "This isn't going to work" or "I can't be bothered to exercise today" or "This is a waste of time."

If you experience this type of resistance, resolutely make yourself do the exercises! Repeat the affirmation "My eyes are getting better and my vision is improving," and don't let negativity or a bad attitude defeat you!

What will happen is that the exercises will quickly energize you and flush out the mental garbage. The negativity will evaporate, usually within a couple of minutes, leaving you feeling positive and with a sense of power and self-control.

The Power Vision Program can open the doors to a better life, so don't just read it and put it away. Now you have the key to better vision, so use it with confidence, knowing that you'll soon see positive results. Diligently exercise your eyes on a regular basis, and you too will enjoy a lifetime of stronger, healthier eyes and naturally improved vision!

SECTION

3

THE
POWER
EXERCISES

These exercises form the dynamic core of the Power Vision Program. They will increase the range and flexibility of your ciliary muscles and extraocular muscles, making them more dynamic and giving them more degrees of freedom.

The exercises will increase your natural focusing ability, improve the coordination of your eyes, and stimulate the nutrient flow in and around your eyes. Do the exercises at your own pace or in time to music or your breathing.

We recommend doing Clocking, Blinking, and Rolling for one minute each. Do the other exercises for two minutes each. You may find it helpful to use a kitchen timer. The basic exercise sequence is:

- Clocking . . . . One minute

- Flexing . . . . .Two minutes

- Blinking . . . . One minute

- Pushups . . . . .Two minutes

- Rolling. . . . . One minute

- Detailing . . . . .Two minutes

- Conducting . . . . .Two minutes

- Biofeedback. . . . . .Two minutes

The most important thing is to learn the exercises and do them correctly. Don't take shortcuts. Practice each exercise a few times until you get the hang of it. You'll probably find that some of the exercises are more effective than others or that you gravitate toward specific exercises. You should go with the flow and do those exercises for longer periods of time. Do more of whatever seems to be working.

The Potentiation Effect

If you do an exercise for a longer period of time, you'll get more improvement than doing it for several shorter periods. For example, nine minutes of Conducting will give you more improvement than three separate periods of three minutes. Likewise, two ten-minute exercise sessions per day will give you about three times as much improvement as a single ten-minute session.

Set yourself the goal of exercising your eyes on a regular basis for 10 minutes a day, preferably 20 minutes. Your eyes may feel sore at first because you are stretching the extraocular muscles. ***If you experience sharp pain or your eyes become unpleasantly sore, you must immediately stop!*** Your goal is to develop smooth, controlled movements, so don't jerk your eyes or overdo things.

Some people may become dizzy or feel like they're starting to get a headache. If that happens, stop and close your eyes. Breathe slowly and deeply until you feel comfortable again; then resume the exercise.

- If you have a minor visual problem and want to return to 20/20 acuity, do the exercises without glasses.

- If you already wear glasses and your vision is getting worse and you want to avoid a stronger prescription, do the exercises with your glasses on.

- If you want to get the maximum improvement and reduce your dependency on glasses, do the exercises with a weaker prescription. These can be old, weaker glasses from previous years, or you can get a weaker prescription from an optometrist.

Loosen Up First

Many people who do a lot of reading or close work suffer from muscular tension in the neck and shoulders. Before starting the exercises, do some stretching to loosen up your neck and shoulders to release any tension that may have accumulated, because this can affect your vision.

Do some neck rolls. Slowly rotate your head. Change direction every few turns. Then do some arm swings. Then reach toward the ceiling with both hands. Push higher with one hand, then the other. Then relax and bend forward and touch the floor.

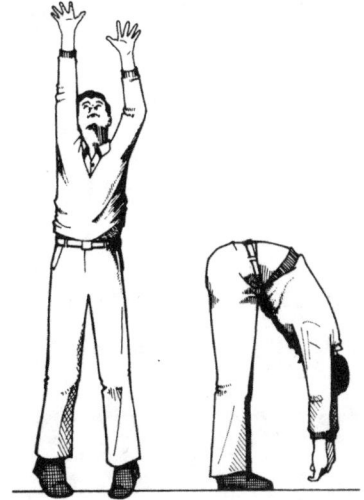

Power Exercise #1: Clocking

What It Is: This important exercise is from India. It's over 2,000 years old and involves looking at the boundaries of your field of vision.

What It Does: Stretches and conditions your extraocular muscles and improves the nutrient flow in and around your eyes.

How to Do It:

Step 1: Breathe slowly and deeply. Look at a far object or something across the room and imagine that you're in front of a giant clock with the far object at the center.

Step 2: Now move your eyes in the 9 o'clock direction as far as they will go as though you're trying to see your left ear. Hold the position for a few seconds with your extraocular muscles fully stretched. Keep your head and neck still by holding your chin if necessary.

Step 3: Now return to the center and look at the far object for a few seconds. Then move your eyes in the 10 o'clock direction, hold for a few seconds, then back to center, then the 11 o'clock direction

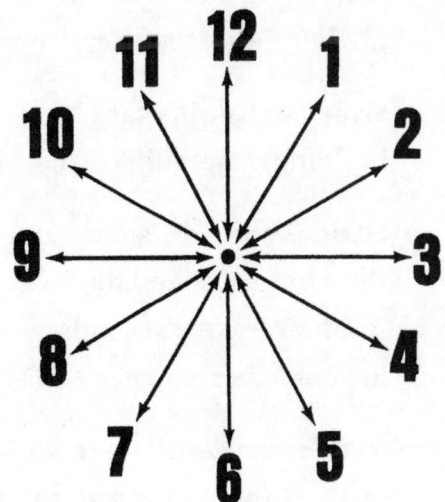

for a few seconds, then back to center. Make your way around the clock, going from the center to each number in turn.

9 > center > 10 > center > 11 > center > 12 > center >1 > center > 2 >...

Carefully stretch your extraocular muscles as far as possible, but not so much that you see flashes of light. Blink every few seconds to keep your eyes lubricated, and aim for smooth, controlled eye movements. When you develop good coordination, do the exercise in time to your breathing:

(inhale / number) > (exhale / center) > (inhale / number) > (exhale / center) >...

Power Exercise #2: Flexing

What It Is: Change focus between a near object and a far object in time to your breathing. Briefly look at a detail on each object every time you change focus.

What It Does: Improves your focusing mechanism and eye muscle coordination. Stimulates the nutrient flow inside your eyes. Increases your natural focusing ability and makes your eyes healthier.

How to Do It:

Step 1: Get a near object with interesting details such as a trinket or piece of jewelry. Don't use anything sharp! You can also use your finger or thumb. Hold the object steady about 6 inches from the tip of your nose. If you hold it farther away, the exercise isn't as effective.

Step 2: Select a far object with details, such as a person, building, automobile, tree, or something across the room.

Step 3: Breathe slowly and deeply. Change focus between the near object and the far object in time to your breathing. Blink every few seconds to keep your eyes lubricated and look at a detail on each object:

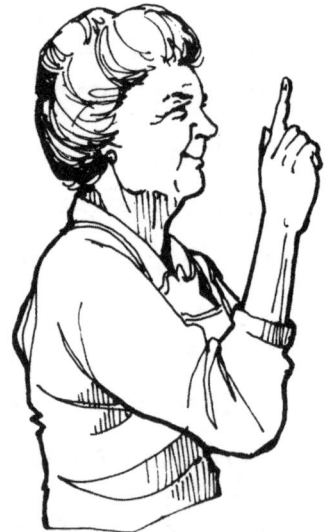

(inhale / near detail) > (exhale / far detail) > (inhale / near detail) > (exhale / far detail) > (inhale / near detail) > (exhale / far detail) > (inhale / near detail) >...

Power Exercise #3: Blinking

What It Is: There are three exercises: Squeeze Blinking, Fast Blinking, and Slow Blinking.

What It Does: Stimulate the flow of nutrients in and around your eyes, making them healthier and stimulating positive changes. The increase in tear fluid may produce a natural contact lens that can improve your acuity and make things clearer.

You can do the exercises without looking at anything in particular, or you can look at details of interesting objects. If you're presbyopic, look at a trinket, or piece of jewelry, or your finger or thumb. If you're myopic, look at a far object such as a tree, building, automobile, person, or something across the room.

The Blinking exercises are so important that you should practice them until they become automatic. They can bring rapid relief from computer vision syndrome and from dry eye disease, and they can help to stop myopia from progressing. Don't do Fast Blinking if you have epilepsy because it may trigger a seizure.

Squeeze Blinking

How to Do It:

Step 1: Gently squeeze your eyes shut using only your eyelid muscles, as though you're gently hugging your eyes with your eyelids. Isolate your eyelid muscles, and don't scrunch up your forehead muscles or the muscles around your eyes.

Ask a friend to watch you and make sure you're doing it correctly. Only use your eyelid muscles. Don't overdo it. The primary purpose is to increase tear fluid production, so a gentle squeeze is all that's needed, not a bear hug!

Step 2: Breathe slowly and deeply. Inhale and look at a detail on an object; then gently squeeze your eyes shut as you exhale:

(inhale / detail) > (exhale / squeeze) > (inhale / detail) > (exhale / squeeze) > . . .

You can do this exercise without looking at anything in particular, in which case the sequence is:

(inhale) > (exhale / squeeze) > (inhale) > (exhale / squeeze) > (inhale) > . . .

Fast Blinking

How to Do It:

Step 1: Breathe slowly and deeply. Inhale and look at a detail on an object; then open and close your eyes as fast as possible as you exhale. Do about a dozen fast blinks every time you exhale. Continue to look at details as you inhale, and fast-blink as you exhale:

(inhale / detail) > (exhale / fast blink) > (inhale / detail) > (exhale / fast blink) > . . .

You can do this exercise without looking at anything in particular, in which case the sequence is:

(inhale) > (exhale / fast blink) > (inhale) > (exhale / fast blink) > (inhale) > . . .

Slow Blinking

How to Do It:

Step 1: Breathe slowly and deeply. Inhale and look at a detail on an object; then gently close your eyes as you exhale. Continue to look at details as you inhale, and gently close your eyes as you exhale:

(inhale / detail) > (exhale / close eyes) > (inhale / detail) > (exhale / close eyes) > . . .

You can do this exercise without looking at anything in particular, in which case the sequence is:

(inhale / open) > (exhale / close) > (inhale / open) > (exhale / close) > . . .

Power Exercise #4: Pushups

What It Is: Also known as *Pencil Pushups*. Hold a pencil at arm's length, or simply look at your thumb. Then slowly move it toward you until you touch the tip of your nose.

What It Does: Increases your focusing ability and improves your eye muscle coordination. Stimulates the nutrient flow inside your eyes and makes your eyes healthier.

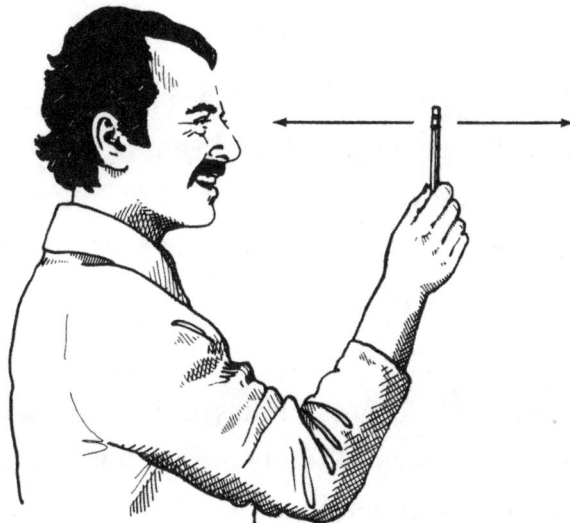

How to Do It:

Step 1: Hold a pencil at arm's length or just use your thumb. You can also use a trinket or piece of jewelry, but don't use anything sharp! Look at a detail such as a letter on the side of the pencil or a wrinkle on your thumb.

Step 2: Breathe slowly and deeply. As you inhale, look at the detail and slowly move the pencil or your thumb toward you until it touches the tip of your nose. Keep looking at the detail and try to maintain a single image at all times.

Step 3: As you exhale, slowly move the pencil or your thumb away to arm's length. Keep looking at the detail and blink every few seconds to keep your eyes lubricated.

(inhale / nose) > (exhale / arm's length) > (inhale / nose) > (exhale /arm's length) > (inhale / nose) > (exhale / arm's length) > (inhale / nose) > . . .

Power Exercise #5: Rolling

What It Is: Slowly roll your eyes in complete or partial circles. Change direction every few seconds.

What It Does: Stretches and conditions your extraocular muscles and improves the nutrient flow in and around your eyes. Makes your eyes healthier and improves the coordination of your extraocular muscles.

How to Do It:

Step 1: Slowly roll your eyes in quarter circles or complete circles, one way, then the other. Keep your head still and hold your chin if necessary. Keep your extraocular muscles fully stretched at all times. Don't overdo it so that you see flashes of light. If you become dizzy, close your eyes and breathe slowly and deeply until the discomfort subsides.

Step 2: In the beginning, take it slow and concentrate on developing good coordination with your extraocular muscles fully stretched. Blink every few seconds to keep your eyes lubricated. Later, when you have good coordination, do the exercise in time to your breathing:

(inhale / clockwise) > (exhale / counterclockwise) > (inhale / clockwise) > (exhale / counterclockwise) > (inhale / clockwise) > (exhale / counterclockwise) > . . .

Power Exercise #6: Detailing

What It Is: Study details by running your gaze along their edges.

What It Does: Improves your eye coordination and sharpens your acuity. This is an important exercise that can quickly open your eyes to a brighter, clearer way of seeing.

How to Do It:

Step 1: Get an interesting object with lots of details, such as a bouquet, trinket, or ornament. Put it at your blur threshold so that some of it is clear but most of it is slightly blurred. If you already see well up close, look at details on a slightly blurred far object. If you can't see well up close, look at details on a slightly blurred near object.

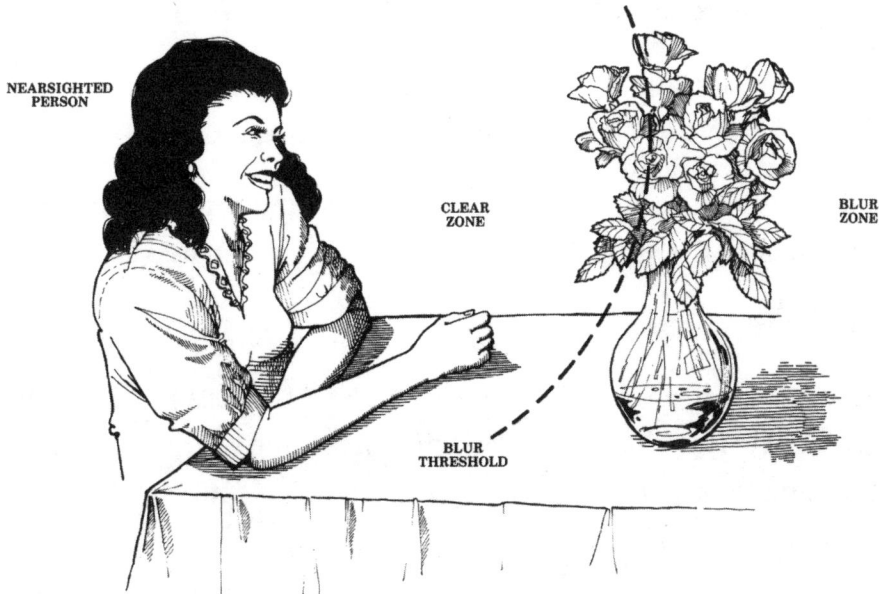

NEARSIGHTED
PERSON

CLEAR
ZONE

BLUR
ZONE

BLUR
THRESHOLD

Step 2: Do a Squeeze Blink, then do a few Fast Blinks, and then run your gaze along the edges of a large detail, such as a leaf if you're using a bouquet. Aim for a calm, contemplative state of mind and briefly study the exact shape of the detail. Don't squint, strain, or try to force yourself to see clearly. This is called the *Clearing Sequence* because it can often clear up slightly blurred images:

Squeeze Blink > Fast Blink > detail

Step 3: Now run your gaze along the edge of a smaller detail inside the detail you are looking at and briefly study its shape, for example, a vein if you're studying a leaf. Then run your gaze along the edge of an even smaller detail and briefly study its shape. Go to the limits of your perception and study the smallest details you can see. As you study the details, remember to blink every few seconds to keep your eyes lubricated.

Alternative Step 3: Try this important variation. Instead of starting with a large detail and progressing to smaller details, do the Clearing Sequence and immediately look at the smallest detail you can see. Run your gaze along its edge and briefly study its shape. You may see even smaller details inside the detail you are looking at, in which case repeat the procedure.

Power Exercise #7: Conducting

What It Is: Look at your thumb or an object in your hand while you slowly make patterns in the space in front of you, like a conductor slowly waving a baton.

What It Does: Increases your focusing ability and improves your eye muscle coordination. Stimulates the nutrient flow inside your eyes and makes your eyes healthier.

How to Do It:

Step 1: Get an object with some interesting details, such as a trinket or piece of jewelry. Or simply use your thumb. Don't use anything sharp! Hold the object at arm's length and look at a detail.

Step 2: Now slowly move your hand. Up, down, back and forth, side to side, circles, diagonals, figure eights, spirals, and even more complex patterns as though you're slowly conducting an orchestra. You can write affirmations in the air, such as "My eyes are getting better and my vision is improving!"

You can do the exercise to music, but don't rush. Concentrate on slow movements with your full attention on the detail. Make patterns from arm's length to the tip of your nose.

Look at the detail at all times and try to maintain a single image as long as possible. Blink every few seconds to keep your eyes lubricated. If your arm gets tired, use the other arm.

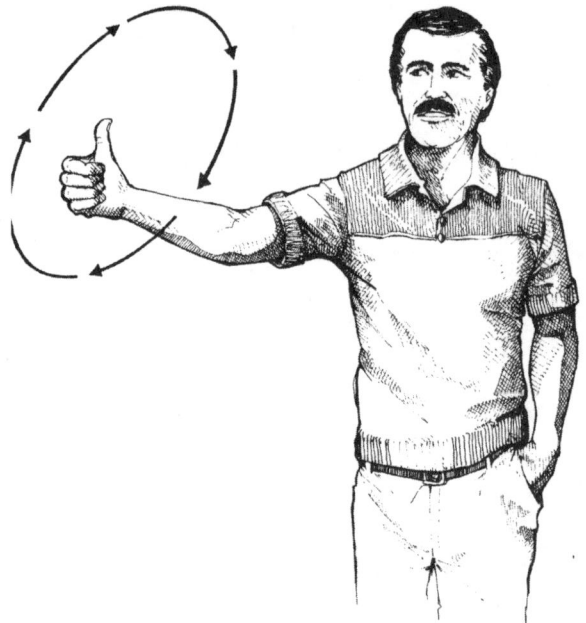

Power Exercise #8: Biofeedback Chart

What It Is: This important exercise can produce a noticeable improvement in acuity, often within a few minutes. In our seminars, many patients were shocked to see the entire chart suddenly become completely clear.

What It Does: Captures the tiny movements your ciliary muscles are constantly making as your eyes try to obtain the sharpest image, and guides your ciliary muscles to form clearer images..

How to Do It: We've provided you with eight charts with different subject matter. Choose the chart you want to work with, and put it where it's slightly blurred with good lighting. Don't hold the chart in your hand. Put it against something solid so it's at a fixed distance.

Now breathe slowly and deeply and do the Clearing Sequence: Squeeze Blink > Fast Blink > detail. Look at the smallest line you can read. It should be slightly blurred but not so blurred that you can't make out the shape of the words. Don't squint, strain, or try to force yourself to see clearly. Aim for a calm, relaxed, contemplative state of mind.

Slowly run your gaze back and forth along the line. Study one of the words and try to make out its shape. Run your gaze along the edges of the word and try to see the individual letters and serifs—the little hooks on the ends of letters. Remember to blink every few seconds to keep your eyes lubricated.

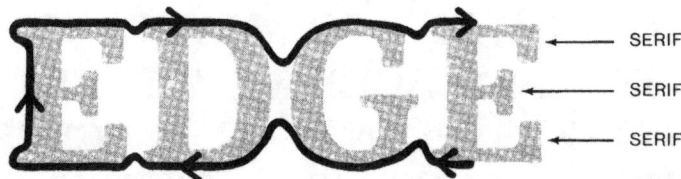

When you can read most of the words on that line, go to the line below, which consists of slightly smaller words, and repeat the exercise. Slowly make your way down the chart to smaller and smaller lines. If the chart suddenly becomes clear, move it to where it is slightly blurred and resume the exercise.

Print extra charts and put them in prominent positions in your home, at work, and in your car. You can use the charts as the near object or the far object for Flexing. Use them as bookmarks. Put one a few pages ahead, and when you reach it, take a break and do the exercise. Experiment and see what works best for you.

Biofeedback Chart A

DEMAND EXCELLENCE! BELIEVE IN YOURSELF AND ANYTHING IS POSSIBLE! GET THE KNOWLEDGE YOU NEED AND USE IT TO YOUR ADVANTAGE! LIVE! LOVE! LAUGH! LEARN TO BE BETTER THAN WHAT YOU ARE! THE SECRET OF GETTING AHEAD IS GETTING STARTED! BE ALL YOU CAN BE! EXCELLENCE IS NOT AN ACT BUT A HABIT! DO IT RIGHT! JUST DO IT! WINNERS MAKE IT HAPPEN! YOU HAVE THE POWER TO MAKE IT HAPPEN! BELIEVE IT AND ACHIEVE IT! LET'S MAKE THINGS BETTER! PLAN FOR SUCCESS! GOOD! BETTER! BEST! SUCCESS IS SWEET! PRACTICE WINNING EVERY DAY! REACH FOR THE STARS! TAKE ADVANTAGE OF THIS OPPORTUNITY! GOD HELPS THOSE WHO HELP THEMSELVES! YOU ARE A WINNER! ATTITUDE IS EVERYTHING! HOPE IS LIKE THE SUN! ENJOY IT! DEDICATION! BECAUSE YOU ARE WORTH IT! TRUST YOUR HIGHER POWER! YOU CAN DO IT! YES YOU CAN! PLAN TO SUCCEED! GET THE WINNING EDGE! DO IT NOW! GO CONFIDENTLY IN THE DIRECTION OF YOUR DREAMS! BELIEVE IT! DO IT! LIVE IT! DO WHATEVER IT TAKES! HIGH PERFORMANCE DELIVERY! THE BEST WAY TO MAKE YOUR DREAMS COME TRUE IS TO WAKE UP! HAVE FUN! ENJOY YOUR LIFE AND DANCE LIKE NOBODY'S WATCHING! AIM HIGH AND SUCCEED! FLY HIGH AND DARE TO DREAM! MAKE IT HAPPEN! REMEMBER, YOU HAVE THE STRENGTH, PATIENCE AND PASSION TO MAKE A DIFFERENCE IN YOUR LIFE! BE BE TRUE, DO YOUR BEST, AND YOU WILL RECEIVE THE HELP YOU NEED! SUCCESS IS THE SUM OF SMALL EFFORTS! FOCUS ON YOUR STRONG POINTS! ONE STEP, ONE DAY AT A TIME! DO RANDOM ACTS OF KINDNESS AND COMPASSION! DEDICATE YOURSELF TO THE GOOD YOU DESERVE AND DESIRE FOR YOURSELF! DANCE BETWEEN THE RAINDROPS! WHERE THERE'S A WILL THERE'S A WAY! CONCENTRATE AND USE YOUR TIME WISELY! TRY TO ACCOMPLISH SOMETHING EVERY DAY! THE FUTURE BELONGS TO THOSE WHO BELIEVE IN THEIR DREAMS! WINNING IS A HABIT! SUCCESS IS A CHOICE YOU MAKE!

Biofeedback Chart B

IN THE HEART OF CITIES, WHERE THE RESTLESS DWELL, AMIDST THE HUSTLE OF LIFE AND TOLLING BELL THERE WALKS A FIGURE, SILENT IN HER GRACE ~ A SEEKER OF TRUTH IN EVERY HIDDEN PLACE. HER EYES, A WINDOW TO THE SOUL'S DELIGHT, PIERCE THE SHADOWS OF THE LONGEST NIGHT. WITH EVERY STEP, SHE DANCES IN THE LIGHT, A RADIANT BEACON IN THE DARKEST NIGHT. SHE MOVES THROUGH HER LIFE WITH WISDOM PURE AND FREE, AND HER MIND IS A WONDROUS TREASURE OF HOPE AND MYSTERY. HER JOYOUS PLAYFUL LAUGHTER NOW CASTS A SPELL ~ BANISHING DARKNESS WHERE DESPAIR MAY DWELL. HER LAUGHTER RINGS LIKE BELLS ON AN ENCHANTED MORNING ~ IN HER, WE SEE THE BEAUTY OF THE HUMAN RACE, A SPIRIT FULL OF LOVE, WHERE THE WEARY FIND THEIR PEACE, AND WITH HER SMILE, ALL BURDENS RELEASE. SHE TREADS THE PATHS WHERE FEW WOULD DARE TO ROAM, HER SPIRIT SHINES, A GUIDE TO LEAD THEM HOME. IN EVERY HEART WHERE DOUBT AND FEAR RESIDE, SHE PLANTS A SEED OF HOPE, A SPARK OF PRIDE. THE WINDS OF CHANGE MAY HOWL AND RAGE ON HIGH, YET IN THEIR MIDST, HER SPIRIT DARES TO FLY. A DREAMER IN A LAND OF ENDLESS GRAY, SHE TURNS THE NIGHT INTO A GLORIOUS DAY. WITH WIT AS SHARP AS A POET'S QUILL, SHE WEAVES HER TALES WITH CHARM, GRACE, AND SKILL. HER WISDOM FLOWS LIKE RIVERS RUNNING FREE, CARRYING THE MESSAGE OF HER LIBERTY. IN FIELDS WHERE FLOWERS BLOOM BENEATH THE SUN SHE GATHERS STRENGTH FROM BATTLES SHE HAS WON. HER JOURNEY, ONE OF COURAGE AND MIGHT, A TESTAMENT OF LOVE'S ENDURING LIGHT. IN HER PRESENCE, DOUBT AND FEAR WILL FLEE, FOR SHE EMBODIES WHAT IT MEANS TO BE FREE. HER JOURNEY AN ODYSSEY OF HEART AND MIND, A PATH OF LOVE THAT LEAVES NO ONE BEHIND, FOR IN HER SOUL, A LIGHT FOREVER SHINES, GUIDING US THROUGH LIFE'S COMPLEX DESIGNS, SO LET US CHERISH THIS BEACON BRIGHT. LET US FOLLOW WHERE HER LIGHT MAY LEAD. EMBRACE THE DREAMS THAT IN OUR HEARTS DO BREED. FOR IN HER WORDS A PROMISE SHINES SO BRIGHT, A FUTURE BATHED IN LOVE AND LIGHT.

Biofeedback Chart C

A MAN STANDS TALL WITH AN UNWAVERING GAZE, LIGHTING THE WORLD IN A MILLION WAYS. HE'S NOT A PRINCE NOR A KING NOR A MAN OF FAME BUT HIS SPIRIT BURNS BRIGHT WITH AN ENDLESS FLAME. WITH HIS HEART OF GOLD AND HANDS OF STEEL, HE SHOWS THE WORLD WHAT IT MEANS TO BE REAL. IN THE PRESENCE OF EVIL HE STANDS HIS GROUND, A PILLAR OF STRENGTH AND LOVE PROFOUND. A MAN OF HONOR, TRUST, AND GRACE, A FRIENDLY SMILE ON HIS RUGGED FACE. FROM DAWN'S FIRST LIGHT TO EVENING'S SHADE, HE WORKS WITH PRIDE IN THE LIFE HE'S MADE. HE FINDS FULFILLMENT AND JOY IN THE SIMPLEST THINGS A BIRD'S SONG AND THE WAY THE WIND SINGS. THE LAUGHTER OF CHILDREN, THE WHISPER OF TREES, IN THE QUIET MOMENTS, HIS SOUL FINDS PEACE. HE'S A FRIEND TO MANY, A STRANGER TO NONE. WITH ARMS WIDE OPEN, HE WELCOMES THE DAWN. HIS KINDNESS FLOWS LIKE A RIVER WIDE, AN ENDLESS SOURCE, A GENTLE PRIDE. FROM HELPING HIS NEIGHBORS TO LENDING A HAND, FROM FIXING A FENCE TO TAKING A STAND. HIS WORDS ARE SIMPLE AND HONEST AND YET THEY HEAL, A WHISPERED TRUTH, A TIMELESS FEEL, AND IN EVERY ACT, HIS VIRTUES GLEAM, A TESTAMENT TO THE AMERICAN DREAM. HE STANDS FOR JUSTICE AND FIGHTS FOR RIGHT, A BEACON OF HOPE IN THE DARKEST NIGHT. WITH COURAGE AND WISDOM, HE SHOWS US THE WAY, INSPIRING OTHERS EVERY DAY. HE SHARES HIS KNOWLEDGE, A GUIDING STAR, HELPING OTHERS NEAR AND FAR. WITH EVERY STORY, WITH EVERY SONG, HE SHOWS THE WORLD WHERE WE BELONG. IN EVERY CHALLENGE HE FINDS GREAT STRENGTH. IN EVERY STRUGGLE HE GOES THE LENGTH. HIS SPIRIT UNBROKEN STANDS PROUD AND TALL, A SYMBOL OF JOY AND HOPE FOR US ALL. THE ROAD AHEAD MAY TWIST AND TURN, BUT HIS STEADY FLAME WILL AWAYS BURN WITH LOYALTY, TRUST, AND HONOR AS HIS GUIDE. HERE'S TO THE MAN WHOSE LIGHT SHINES BRIGHT, INSPIRING OTHERS DAY AND NIGHT. HE IS TRUE TO HIMSELF, AND IN EVERY STEP, A TALE UNFOLDS, A STORY FOREVER TO BE TOLD. AS THE SUN SETS AND THE MOON ASCENDS, HIS JOURNEY CONTINUES AND HIS LEGACY EXTENDS.

Biofeedback Chart D

FOR GOD SO LOVED THE WORLD, THAT HE GAVE HIS ONLY BEGOTTEN SON, THAT WHOSOVER BELIEVETH IN HIM SHOULD NOT PERISH, BUT HAVE EVERLASTING LIFE. FOR GOD SENT HIS SON INTO THE WORLD NOT TO CONDEMN THE WORLD, BUT THAT THE WORLD THROUGH HIM MIGHT BE SAVED. HE THAT BELIEVETH ON HIM IS NOT CONDEMNED, BUT HE THAT BELIEVETH NOT IS CONDEMNED ALREADY BECAUSE HE HATH NOT BELIEVED IN THE NAME OF THE ONLY BEGOTTEN SON OF GOD. AND THIS IS THE CONDEMNATION, THAT LIGHT IS COME INTO THE WORLD, AND MEN LOVED DARKNESS RATHER THAN LIGHT, BECAUSE THEIR DEEDS WERE EVIL. FOR EVERYONE THAT DOETH EVIL HATETH THE LIGHT, NEITHER COMETH TO THE LIGHT, LEST HIS DEEDS SHOULD BE REPROVED. BUT HE THAT DOETH TRUTH COMETH TO THE LIGHT, THAT HIS DEEDS MAY BE MANIFEST, THAT THEY ARE WROUGHT IN GOD. AFTER THESE THINGS CAME JESUS AND HIS DISCIPLES INTO THE LAND OF JUDAEA, AND THERE HE TARRIED WITH THEM AND BAPTIZED. AND JOHN WAS ALSO BAPTIZING IN AENON NEAR TO SALIM, BECAUSE THERE WAS MUCH WATER THERE, AND WERE BAPTIZED. FOR JOHN WAS NOT YET CAST INTO PRISON. THEN THERE AROSE A QUESTION BETWEEN SOME OF JOHN'S DISCIPLES AND THE JEWS ABOUT PURIFYING. AND THEY CAME UNTO JOHN, AND SAID UNTO HIM, RABBI, HE THAT WAS WITH THEE BEYOND JORDAN, WHOM THOU BARE WITNESS, BEHOLD, THE SAME BAPTIZETH, AND ALL MEN COME TO HIM. JOHN ANSWERED AND SAID, A MAN CAN RECEIVE NOTHING, EXCEPT IT BE GIVEN HIM FROM HEAVEN. YE YOURSELVES BEAR ME WITNESS, THAT I SAID, I AM NOT THE CHRIST, BUT THAT I AM SENT BEFORE HIM. HE THAT HATH THE BRIDE IS THE BRIDGROOM, BUT THE FRIEND OF THE BRIDEGROOM, WHICH STANDETH AND HEARETH HIM, REJOICETH GREATLY BECAUSE OF THE BRIDGROOM'S VOICE. THIS MY JOY THEREFORE IS FULFILLED. HE MUST INCREASE, BUT I MUST DECREASE. HE THAT COMETH FROM

Biofeedback Chart E

CONGRESS SHALL MAKE NO LAW RESPECTING AN ESTABLISHMENT OF RELIGION, OR PROHIBITING THE FREE EXERCISE THEREOF, OR ABRIDGING THE FREEDOM OF SPEECH, OR OF THE PRESS, OR THE RIGHT OF THE PEOPLE TO PEACEABLY ASSEMBLE AND TO PETITION CONGRESS FOR A REDRESS OF GRIEVANCES. A WELL REGULATED MILITIA, BEING NECESSARY TO THE SECURITY OF A FREE STATE, THE RIGHT OF THE PEOPLE TO KEEP AND BEAR ARMS SHALL NOT BE INFRINGED. NO SOLDIER SHALL, IN TIME OF PEACE, BE QUARTERED IN ANY HOUSE WITHOUT THE CONSENT OF THE OWNER, NOR IN TIME OF WAR, BUT IN A MANNER TO BE PRESCRIBED BY LAW. THE RIGHT OF THE PEOPLE TO BE SECURE IN THEIR PERSONS, HOUSES, PAPERS, AND EFFECTS, AGAINST UNREASONABLE SEARCHES AND SEIZURES, SHALL NOT BE VIOLATED, AND NO WARRANTS SHALL ISSUE, BUT UPON PROBABLE CAUSE, SUPPORTED BY OATH OR AFFIRMATION, AND PARTICULARLY DESCRIBING THE PLACE TO BE SEARCHED, AND THE PERSONS OR THINGS TO BE SEIZED. NO PERSON SHALL BE HELD TO ANSWER FOR A CAPITAL OR OTHERWISE INFAMOUS CRIME, UNLESS ON A PRESENTMENT OR INDICTMENT OF A GRAND JURY, EXCEPT IN CASES ARISING IN THE LAND OR NAVAL FORCES, OR IN THE MILITIA, WHEN IN ACTUAL SERVICE IN TIME OF WAR OR PUBLIC DANGER, NOR SHALL ANY PERSON BE SUBJECT FOR THE SAME OFFENCE TO BE TWICE PUT IN JEOPARDY OF LIFE OR LIMB, NOR SHALL BE COMPELLED IN ANY CRIMINAL CASE TO BE A WITNESS AGAINST HIMSELF, NOR BE DEPRIVED OF LIFE, LIBERTY, OR PROPERTY, WITHOUT DUE PROCESS OF LAW, NOR SHALL PROPERTY BE TAKEN FOR PUBLIC USE, WITHOUT JUST COMPENSATION. IN ALL CRIMINAL PROSECUTIONS, THE ACCUSED SHALL ENJOY THE RIGHT TO A SPEEDY AND PUBLIC TRIAL, BY AN IMPARTIAL JURY OF THE STATE AND DISTRICT WHEREIN THE CRIME SHALL HAVE BEEN COMMITTED, WHICH DISTRICT SHALL HAVE BEEN PREVIOUSLY ASCERTAINED BY LAW, AND TO BE INFORMED OF THE

Biofeedback Chart F

A CLEAR CONSCIENCE IS A SIGN OF A BAD MEMORY. TWO WRONGS DON'T MAKE A RIGHT, BUT THEY MAKE A GOOD EXCUSE. ONE LOYAL FRIEND IS BETTER THAN A THOUSAND RELATIVES. EXPERIENCE IS SIMPLY THE NAME WE GIVE OUR MISTAKES. ALL YOU NEED IS LOVE, BUT A LITTLE CHOCOLATE DOESN'T HURT. IT'S USELESS TO HOLD A MAN TO ANYTHING HE SAYS WHEN HE'S DRUNK, MADLY IN LOVE, OR RUNNING FOR CONGRESS. WOMEN ARE MADE TO BE LOVED, NOT UNDERSTOOD. IF YOU THINK MONEY CAN'T BUY YOU HAPPINESS, YOU DON'T KNOW WHERE TO GO SHOPPING. GRANDPARENTS SPRINKLE STARDUST OVER THE LIVES OF LITTLE CHILDREN. THERE ARE THREE KINDS OF PEOPLE, THOSE WHO CAN DO MATH AND THOSE WHO CAN'T. REST ASSURED THAT IN REAL LIFE, THERE IS NO SUCH THING AS ALGEBRA. ALWAYS FORGIVE YOUR ENEMIES, NOTHING ANNOYS THEM SO MUCH. IF YOU CAN'T BE KIND, AT LEAST BE VAGUE. IT'S ABSURD TO DIVIDE PEOPLE INTO GOOD OR BAD ~ PEOPLE ARE EITHER CHARMING OR TEDIOUS. WHEN YOUR FRIENDS FLATTER YOU ON HOW YOUNG YOU LOOK, IT'S A SURE SIGN THAT YOU'RE GETTING OLD. THE DIFFERENCE BETWEEN GENIUS AND STUPIDITY IS THAT GENIUS HAS ITS LIMITS. ON THE WHOLE, PEOPLE WANT TO BE GOOD BUT NOT TOO GOOD AND NOT ALL THE TIME. LIFE IS NEVER FAIR, AND PERHAPS IT IS A GOOD THING THAT IT IS NOT. BEHIND EVERY GREAT MAN IS A WOMAN ROLLING HER EYES. PEOPLE WHO THINK THEY KNOW EVERYTHING ARE AN ANNOYANCE TO THOSE OF US WHO DO. AGE IS AN ISSUE OF MIND OVER MATTER. IF YOU DON'T MIND IT DOESN'T MATTER. THE BEST THING ABOUT THE FUTURE IS THAT IT COMES ONE DAY AT A TIME. THE ONLY THING WORSE THAN BEING TALKED ABOUT IS NOT BEING TALKED ABOUT. A STEADY INCOME IS BETTER THAN A REPUTATION FOR BEING BRILLIANT. IT TAKES CONSIDERABLE KNOWLEDGE TO REALIZE THE EXTENT OF ONE'S IGNORANCE. GET YOUR FACTS FIRST, THEN YOU CAN DISTORT THEM AS YOU PLEASE. DON'T ARGUE, JUST EXPLAIN WHY YOU'RE RIGHT. ALWAYS REMEMBER THAT YOU'RE UNIQUE, JUST LIKE EVERYONE ELSE. I CAN RESIST EVERYTHING EXCEPT TEMPTATION.

Biofeedback Chart G

O NOBLE GUARDIAN OF MY HEART IN TWILIGHT'S HUSH, WHERE DREAMS AND SHADOWS BLEND, THY VISAGE SHINES, MY TRULY FAITHFUL FRIEND. WITH RUGGED GRACE THY FORM DOTH PROUDLY STAND, A BASTION FIRM, BOTH GENTLE AND YET GRAND. THINE EYES LIKE ORBS OF DEEPEST BLUE, REFLECT THE SKIES ~ ETERNAL, VAST, AND TRUE. THY BROW IS MARKED WITH WISDOM'S NOBLE TRACE, EACH LINE A TESTAMENT TO STRENGTH AND GRACE. WITH COURAGE SUBLIME, THOU MEETEST THE RISING SUN. A A WARRIOR FIERCE ~ YET KIND TO EVERYONE. THY VOICE, A MELODY SO RICH AND RARE, DOTH WEAVE A CHARM BEYOND COMPARE. O MAN OF VIRTUE, COURAGE, TRUTH, AND MIGHT, THY HUMBLE PRESENCE CASTS AWAY THE DARKEST NIGHT. WITH TENDER CARE, THY HANDS BOTH STRONG AND FAIR, LIFT ME HIGH AND BANISH MY DESPAIR. THY NOBLE ARMS, A FORTRESS AGAINST THE STORM OF LIFE'S FIERCE CRY, DO SHELTER ME BENEATH THE STARRY SKY. O GALLANT KNIGHT OF CHIVALROUS DEED, THY VIRTUE RADIANT AND BRIGHT, DOTH DOTH SET MY SOUL AFLAME WITH PASSIONATE DELIGHT. TO THEE, MY SOUL'S ETERNAL GUIDE, MY LOVE, MY FRIEND, MY JOY, MY PRIDE, WITH GRATITUDE MY HEART DOTH SING, O NOBLE GUARDIAN, MY EVERYTHING. THY COURAGE LIKE THE LION'S MIGHTY ROAR, DEFENDS THE WEAK, AND OPENS EVERY DOOR. IN TIMES OF TRIAL, THOU STANDEST PROUD AND TALL. THY HANDS, STRENGTHENED BY UNENDING TOIL, YET GENTLY TOUCH ~ IN LOVE'S SWEET TURMOIL. THEY CRADLE DREAMS AND BANISH SORROW'S FROWN, WITH EVERY TOUCH, THOU WEAREST LOVE'S BRIGHT CROWN. O NOBLE KNIGHT, MY GUARDIAN AND MY FRIEND, IN THEE, MY HEART SHALL EVERMORE DEPEND. FOR IN THY LOVE, I FIND MY TRUEST SELF. WITH THEE, MY SOUL IS FILLED WITH BOUNDLESS WEALTH. THY SPIRIT, NOBLE, VALIANT AND BOLD, A TALE OF HONOR, TIME AND AGAIN RETOLD. THY HEART, A TREASURE RARE AND PURE, OF LOVE UNYIELDING, STEADFAST AND SURE. WITH EVERY BREATH, IN AWE I STAND, A HUMBLE WITNESS TO THY GENTLE HAND. LOVE AND HONOR INTERTWINE, A PERFECT PORTRAIT OF THY SOUL DIVINE.

Biofeedback Chart H

IN THE LABYRINTH OF CITY LIGHTS I FOUND YOU ~ MY SERENE SERENADE. YOUR PRESENCE IS MY FAVORITE SONG ~ A MELODY THAT DANCES IN MY BLOOD, AWAKENING DREAMS LONG BURIED. YOUR LAUGHTER IS THE SUN BREAKING THROUGH THE STORM CLOUDS IN MY MIND, A BLISSFUL WARMTH THAT MELTS AWAY MY FEARS AND MAKES THE WORLD SEEM ALRIGHT AGAIN. TOGETHER, WE'RE WEAVING PRECIOUS MOMENTS INTO ETERNITY. EVERY WHISPERED SECRET, EVERY STOLEN GLANCE, IS A SACRED VOW SEALED IN THE LANGUAGE ONLY OUR HEARTS UNDERSTAND. OUR SOULS CONVERSE IN SILENCE, AND IN THE SPACES BETWEEN WORDS ~ WHERE LOVE SPEAKS THE LOUDEST, IN YOUR ARMS, I'VE FOUND MY TRUE HOME. YOU ARE THE CALM IN MY CHAOS, THE CERTAINTY IN MY MIND, THE BLESSED LOVE I THOUGHT I'D NEVER FIND. YOU ARE MY UNWRITTEN STORY, THE MUSE TO EVERY SONG UNSUNG. WITH YOU, THE MUNDANE BECOMES MAGICAL, EVERYDAY MOMENTS ETCHED INTO THE CANVAS OF MY HEART. YOU ARE THE REASON BEHIND MY SMILES, THE STRENGTH IN MY WEAK MOMENTS, MY PARTNER, MY LOVER, MY BEST FRIEND. IN YOUR SWEET EMBRACE, I FIND A SACRED SANCTUARY WHERE I CAN CAST ASIDE MY MASK AND TRULY BE MYSELF. YOU ARE MY HARBOR, MY REFUGE, THE ONE WHO TRULY SEES ME AND LOVES ME FOR ALL THAT I AM, AND ALL THAT I HOPE TO BE. EACH DAY WITH YOU IS A NEW CHAPTER, A STORY OF LOVE, RESILIENCE, AND HOPE. YOU INSPIRE ME TO DREAM BIGGER, REACH HIGHER, AND LOVE DEEPER. IN YOUR LOVE, I'VE FOUND MY ANCHOR, THE FORCE THAT KEEPS ME STEADY, EVEN WHEN LIFE'S WAVES THREATEN TO KNOCK ME DOWN. YOU ARE MY FOREVER, THE ONE I CHOOSE AGAIN AND AGAIN, IN THIS LIFE AND BEYOND. YOUR LOVE IS A PRECIOUS GIFT I CHERISH, A TREASURE I HOLD DEAR, A BEACON OF LIGHT IN A WORLD SO TREACHEROUS AND DARK. IN YOU, I'VE FOUND MY PERFECT IMPERFECT, A LOVE THAT'S REAL, SUBLIME, AND BEAUTIFUL. I VOW TO LOVE YOU TODAY, TOMORROW, AND ALWAYS, WITH ALL THAT I AM, AND ALL THAT I HOPE TO BE. TOGETHER, WE ARE A FORCE OF NATURE, A SYMPHONY OF LOVE AND LIGHT THAT ASCENDS TO THE REALM OF THE DIVINE.

Biofeedback Chart A

DEMAND EXCELLENCE! BELIEVE IN YOURSELF AND ANYTHING IS POSSIBLE! GET THE KNOWLEDGE YOU NEED AND USE IT TO YOUR ADVANTAGE! LIVE! LOVE! LAUGH! LEARN TO BE BETTER THAN WHAT YOU ARE! THE SECRET OF GETTING AHEAD IS GETTING STARTED! BE ALL YOU CAN BE! EXCELLENCE IS NOT AN ACT BUT A HABIT! DO IT RIGHT! JUST DO IT! WINNERS MAKE IT HAPPEN! YOU HAVE THE POWER TO MAKE IT HAPPEN! BELIEVE IT AND ACHIEVE IT! LET'S MAKE THINGS BETTER! PLAN FOR SUCCESS! GOOD! BETTER! BEST! SUCCESS IS SWEET! PRACTICE WINNING EVERY DAY! REACH FOR THE STARS! TAKE ADVANTAGE OF THIS OPPORTUNITY! GOD HELPS THOSE WHO HELP THEMSELVES! YOU ARE A WINNER! ATTITUDE IS EVERYTHING! HOPE IS LIKE THE SUN! ENJOY IT! DEDICATION! BECAUSE YOU ARE WORTH IT! TRUST YOUR HIGHER POWER! YOU CAN DO IT! YES YOU CAN! PLAN TO SUCCEED! GET THE WINNING EDGE! DO IT NOW! GO CONFIDENTLY IN THE DIRECTION OF YOUR DREAMS! BELIEVE IT! DO IT! LIVE IT! DO WHATEVER IT TAKES! HIGH PERFORMANCE DELIVERY! THE BEST WAY TO MAKE YOUR DREAMS COME TRUE IS TO WAKE UP! HAVE FUN! ENJOY YOUR LIFE AND DANCE LIKE NOBODY'S WATCHING! AIM HIGH AND SUCCEED! FLY HIGH AND DARE TO DREAM! MAKE IT HAPPEN! REMEMBER, YOU HAVE THE STRENGTH, PATIENCE AND PASSION TO MAKE A DIFFERENCE IN YOUR LIFE! BE BE TRUE, DO YOUR BEST, AND YOU WILL RECEIVE THE HELP YOU NEED! SUCCESS IS THE SUM OF SMALL EFFORTS! FOCUS ON YOUR STRONG POINTS! ONE STEP, ONE DAY AT A TIME! DO RANDOM ACTS OF KINDNESS AND COMPASSION! DEDICATE YOURSELF TO THE GOOD YOU DESERVE AND DESIRE FOR YOURSELF! DANCE BETWEEN THE RAINDROPS! WHERE THERE'S A WILL, THERE'S A WAY! CONCENTRATE AND USE YOUR TIME WISELY! TRY TO ACCOMPLISH SOMETHING EVERY DAY! THE FUTURE BELONGS TO THOSE WHO BELIEVE IN THEIR DREAMS! WINNING IS A HABIT! SUCCESS IS A CHOICE YOU MAKE!

Biofeedback Chart B

IN THE HEART OF CITIES, WHERE THE RESTLESS DWELL, AMIDST THE HUSTLE OF LIFE AND TOLLING BELL THERE WALKS A FIGURE, SILENT IN HER GRACE ~ A SEEKER OF TRUTH IN EVERY HIDDEN PLACE. HER EYES, A WINDOW TO THE SOUL'S DELIGHT, PIERCE THE SHADOWS OF THE LONGEST NIGHT. WITH EVERY STEP, SHE DANCES IN THE LIGHT, A RADIANT BEACON IN THE DARKEST NIGHT. SHE MOVES THROUGH HER LIFE WITH WISDOM PURE AND FREE, AND HER MIND IS A WONDROUS TREASURE OF HOPE AND MYSTERY. HER JOYOUS PLAYFUL LAUGHTER NOW CASTS A SPELL ~ BANISHING DARKNESS WHERE DESPAIR MAY DWELL. HER LAUGHTER RINGS LIKE BELLS ON AN ENCHANTED MORNING ~ IN HER, WE SEE THE BEAUTY OF THE HUMAN RACE, A SPIRIT FULL OF LOVE, WHERE THE WEARY FIND THEIR PEACE, AND WITH HER SMILE, ALL BURDENS RELEASE. SHE TREADS THE PATHS WHERE FEW WOULD DARE TO ROAM, HER SPIRIT SHINES, A GUIDE TO LEAD THEM HOME. IN EVERY HEART WHERE DOUBT AND FEAR RESIDE, SHE PLANTS A SEED OF HOPE, A SPARK OF PRIDE. THE WINDS OF CHANGE MAY HOWL AND RAGE ON HIGH, YET IN THEIR MIDST, HER SPIRIT DARES TO FLY. A DREAMER IN A LAND OF ENDLESS GRAY, SHE TURNS THE NIGHT INTO A GLORIOUS DAY. WITH WIT AS SHARP AS A POET'S QUILL, SHE WEAVES HER TALES WITH CHARM, GRACE, AND SKILL. HER WISDOM FLOWS LIKE RIVERS RUNNING FREE, CARRYING THE MESSAGE OF HER LIBERTY. IN FIELDS WHERE FLOWERS BLOOM BENEATH THE SUN SHE GATHERS STRENGTH FROM BATTLES SHE HAS WON. HER JOURNEY, ONE OF COURAGE AND MIGHT, A TESTAMENT OF LOVE'S ENDURING LIGHT. IN HER PRESENCE, DOUBT AND FEAR WILL FLEE, FOR SHE EMBODIES WHAT IT MEANS TO BE FREE. HER JOURNEY AN ODYSSEY OF HEART AND MIND, A PATH OF LOVE THAT LEAVES NO ONE BEHIND, FOR IN HER SOUL, A LIGHT FOREVER SHINES, GUIDING US THROUGH LIFE'S COMPLEX DESIGNS. SO LET US CHERISH THIS BEACON BRIGHT, LET US FOLLOW WHERE HER LIGHT MAY LEAD. EMBRACE THE DREAMS THAT IN OUR HEARTS DO BREED. FOR IN HER WORDS A PROMISE SHINES SO BRIGHT, A FUTURE BATHED IN LOVE AND LIGHT.

Biofeedback Chart C

A MAN STANDS TALL WITH AN UNWAVERING GAZE, LIGHTING THE WORLD IN A MILLION WAYS. HE'S NOT A PRINCE NOR A KING NOR A MAN OF FAME BUT HIS SPIRIT BURNS BRIGHT WITH AN ENDLESS FLAME. WITH HIS HEART OF GOLD AND HANDS OF STEEL, HE SHOWS THE WORLD WHAT IT MEANS TO BE REAL. IN THE PRESENCE OF EVIL HE STANDS HIS GROUND, A PILLAR OF STRENGTH AND LOVE PROFOUND. A MAN OF HONOR, TRUST, AND GRACE, A FRIENDLY SMILE ON HIS RUGGED FACE. FROM DAWN'S FIRST LIGHT TO EVENING'S SHADE, HE WORKS WITH PRIDE IN THE LIFE HE'S MADE. HE FINDS FULFILLMENT AND JOY IN THE SIMPLEST THINGS A BIRD'S SONG AND THE WAY THE WIND SINGS. THE LAUGHTER OF CHILDREN, THE WHISPER OF TREES, IN THE QUIET MOMENTS, HIS SOUL FINDS PEACE. HE'S A FRIEND TO MANY, A STRANGER TO NONE. WITH ARMS WIDE OPEN, HE WELCOMES THE DAWN. HIS KINDNESS FLOWS LIKE A RIVER WIDE, AN ENDLESS SOURCE, A GENTLE PRIDE. FROM HELPING HIS NEIGHBORS TO LENDING A HAND, FROM FIXING A FENCE TO TAKING A STAND. HIS WORDS ARE SIMPLE AND HONEST AND YET THEY HEAL, A WHISPERED TRUTH, A TIMELESS FEEL, AND IN EVERY ACT, HIS VIRTUES GLEAM, A TESTAMENT TO THE AMERICAN DREAM. HE STANDS FOR JUSTICE AND FIGHTS FOR RIGHT, A BEACON OF HOPE IN THE DARKEST NIGHT. WITH COURAGE AND WISDOM, HE SHOWS US THE WAY, INSPIRING OTHERS EVERY DAY. HE SHARES HIS KNOWLEDGE, A GUIDING STAR, HELPING OTHERS NEAR AND FAR. WITH EVERY STORY, WITH EVERY SONG, HE SHOWS THE WORLD WHERE WE BELONG. IN EVERY CHALLENGE HE FINDS GREAT STRENGTH. IN EVERY STRUGGLE HE GOES THE LENGTH. HIS SPIRIT UNBROKEN STANDS PROUD AND TALL, A SYMBOL OF JOY AND HOPE FOR US ALL. THE ROAD AHEAD MAY TWIST AND TURN, BUT HIS STEADY FLAME WILL ALWAYS BURN WITH LOYALTY, TRUST, AND HONOR AS HIS GUIDE. HERE'S TO THE MAN WHOSE LIGHT SHINES BRIGHT, INSPIRING OTHERS DAY AND NIGHT. HE IS TRUE TO HIMSELF, AND IN EVERY STEP, A TALE UNFOLDS, A STORY FOREVER TO BE TOLD. AS THE SUN SETS AND THE MOON ASCENDS, HIS JOURNEY CONTINUES AND HIS LEGACY EXTENDS.

Biofeedback Chart D

FOR GOD SO LOVED THE WORLD, THAT HE GAVE HIS ONLY BEGOTTEN SON, THAT WHOSOVER BELIEVETH IN HIM SHOULD NOT PERISH, BUT HAVE EVERLASTING LIFE. FOR GOD SENT HIS SON INTO THE WORLD NOT TO CONDEMN THE WORLD, BUT THAT THE WORLD THROUGH HIM MIGHT BE SAVED. HE THAT BELIEVETH ON HIM IS NOT CONDEMNED, BUT HE THAT BELIEVETH NOT IS CONDEMNED ALREADY BECAUSE HE HATH NOT BELIEVED IN THE NAME OF THE ONLY BEGOTTEN SON OF GOD. AND THIS IS THE CONDEMNATION, THAT LIGHT IS COME INTO THE WORLD, AND MEN LOVED DARKNESS RATHER THAN LIGHT, BECAUSE THEIR DEEDS WERE EVIL. FOR EVERYONE THAT DOETH EVIL HATETH THE LIGHT, NEITHER COMETH TO THE LIGHT, LEST HIS DEEDS SHOULD BE REPROVED. BUT HE THAT DOETH TRUTH COMETH TO THE LIGHT, THAT HIS DEEDS MAY BE MANIFEST, THAT THEY ARE WROUGHT IN GOD. AFTER THESE THINGS CAME JESUS AND HIS DISCIPLES INTO THE LAND OF JUDAEA, AND THERE HE TARRIED WITH THEM AND BAPTIZED. AND JOHN WAS ALSO BAPTIZING IN AENON NEAR TO SALIM, BECAUSE THERE WAS MUCH WATER THERE, AND WERE BAPTIZED. FOR JOHN WAS NOT YET CAST INTO PRISON. THEN THERE AROSE A QUESTION BETWEEN SOME OF JOHN'S DISCIPLES AND THE JEWS ABOUT PURIFYING. AND THEY CAME UNTO JOHN, AND SAID UNTO HIM, RABBI, HE THAT WAS WITH THEE BEYOND JORDAN, WHOM THOU BARE WITNESS, BEHOLD, THE SAME BAPTIZETH, AND ALL MEN COME TO HIM. JOHN ANSWERED AND SAID, A MAN CAN RECEIVE NOTHING, EXCEPT IT BE GIVEN HIM FROM HEAVEN. YE YOURSELVES BEAR ME WITNESS, THAT I SAID, I AM NOT THE CHRIST, BUT THAT I AM SENT BEFORE HIM. HE THAT HATH THE BRIDE IS THE BRIDEGROOM. BUT THE FRIEND OF THE BRIDEGROOM, WHICH STANDETH AND HEARETH HIM, REJOICETH GREATLY BECAUSE OF THE BRIDEGROOM'S VOICE. THIS MY JOY THEREFORE IS FULFILLED. HE MUST INCREASE, BUT I MUST DECREASE. HE THAT COMETH FROM

Biofeedback Chart E

CONGRESS SHALL MAKE NO LAW RESPECTING AN ESTABLISHMENT OF RELIGION, OR PROHIBITING THE FREE EXERCISE THEREOF, OR ABRIDGING THE FREEDOM OF SPEECH, OR OF THE PRESS, OR THE RIGHT OF THE PEOPLE TO PEACEABLY ASSEMBLE AND TO PETITION CONGRESS FOR A REDRESS OF GRIEVANCES. A WELL REGULATED MILITIA, BEING NECESSARY TO THE SECURITY OF A FREE STATE, THE RIGHT OF THE PEOPLE TO KEEP AND BEAR ARMS SHALL NOT BE INFRINGED. NO SOLDIER SHALL, IN TIME OF PEACE, BE QUARTERED IN ANY HOUSE WITHOUT THE CONSENT OF THE OWNER, NOR IN TIME OF WAR, BUT IN A MANNER TO BE PRESCRIBED BY LAW. THE RIGHT OF THE PEOPLE TO BE SECURE IN THEIR PERSONS, HOUSES, PAPERS, AND EFFECTS, AGAINST UNREASONABLE SEARCHES AND SEIZURES, SHALL NOT BE VIOLATED, AND NO WARRANTS SHALL ISSUE, BUT UPON PROBABLE CAUSE, SUPPORTED BY OATH OR AFFIRMATION, AND PARTICULARLY DESCRIBING THE PLACE TO BE SEARCHED, AND THE PERSONS OR THINGS TO BE SEIZED. NO PERSON SHALL BE HELD TO ANSWER FOR A CAPITAL OR OTHERWISE INFAMOUS CRIME, UNLESS ON A PRESENTMENT OR INDICTMENT OF A GRAND JURY, EXCEPT IN CASES ARISING IN THE LAND OR NAVAL FORCES, OR IN THE MILITIA, WHEN IN ACTUAL SERVICE IN TIME OF WAR OR PUBLIC DANGER. NOR SHALL ANY PERSON BE SUBJECT FOR THE SAME OFFENCE TO BE TWICE PUT IN JEOPARDY OF LIFE OR LIMB. NOR SHALL BE COMPELLED IN ANY CRIMINAL CASE TO BE A WITNESS AGAINST HIMSELF, NOR BE DEPRIVED OF LIFE, LIBERTY, OR PROPERTY, WITHOUT DUE PROCESS OF LAW. NOR SHALL PROPERTY BE TAKEN FOR PUBLIC USE, WITHOUT JUST COMPENSATION. IN ALL CRIMINAL PROSECUTIONS, THE ACCUSED SHALL ENJOY THE RIGHT TO A SPEEDY AND PUBLIC TRIAL, BY AN IMPARTIAL JURY OF THE STATE AND DISTRICT WHEREIN THE CRIME SHALL HAVE BEEN COMMITTED, WHICH DISTRICT SHALL HAVE BEEN PREVIOUSLY ASCERTAINED BY LAW, AND TO BE INFORMED OF THE

Biofeedback Chart F

A CLEAR CONSCIENCE IS A SIGN OF A BAD MEMORY. TWO WRONGS DON'T MAKE A RIGHT, BUT THEY MAKE A GOOD EXCUSE. ONE LOYAL FRIEND IS BETTER THAN A THOUSAND RELATIVES. EXPERIENCE IS SIMPLY THE NAME WE GIVE OUR MISTAKES. ALL YOU NEED IS LOVE, BUT A LITTLE CHOCOLATE DOESN'T HURT. IT'S USELESS TO HOLD A MAN TO ANYTHING HE SAYS WHEN HE'S DRUNK, MADLY IN LOVE, OR RUNNING FOR CONGRESS. WOMEN ARE MADE TO BE LOVED, NOT UNDERSTOOD. IF YOU THINK MONEY CAN'T BUY YOU HAPPINESS, YOU DON'T KNOW WHERE TO GO SHOPPING. GRANDPARENTS SPRINKLE STARDUST OVER THE LIVES OF LITTLE CHILDREN. THERE ARE THREE KINDS OF PEOPLE, THOSE WHO CAN DO MATH AND THOSE WHO CAN'T. REST ASSURED THAT IN REAL LIFE, THERE IS NO SUCH THING AS ALGEBRA. ALWAYS FORGIVE YOUR ENEMIES, NOTHING ANNOYS THEM SO MUCH. IF YOU CAN'T BE KIND, AT LEAST BE VAGUE. IT'S ABSURD TO DIVIDE PEOPLE INTO GOOD OR BAD ~ PEOPLE ARE EITHER CHARMING OR TEDIOUS. WHEN YOUR FRIENDS FLATTER YOU ON HOW YOUNG YOU LOOK, IT'S A SURE SIGN THAT YOU'RE GETTING OLD. THE DIFFERENCE BETWEEN GENIUS AND STUPIDITY IS THAT GENIUS HAS ITS LIMITS. ON THE WHOLE, PEOPLE WANT TO BE GOOD BUT NOT TOO GOOD AND NOT ALL THE TIME. LIFE IS NEVER FAIR, AND PERHAPS IT IS A GOOD THING THAT IT IS NOT. BEHIND EVERY GREAT MAN IS A WOMAN ROLLING HER EYES. PEOPLE WHO THINK THEY KNOW EVERYTHING ARE AN ANNOYANCE TO THOSE OF US WHO DO. AGE IS AN ISSUE OF MIND OVER MATTER. IF YOU DON'T MIND IT DOESN'T MATTER. THE BEST THING ABOUT THE FUTURE IS THAT IT COMES ONE DAY AT A TIME. THE ONLY THING WORSE THAN BEING TALKED ABOUT IS NOT BEING TALKED ABOUT. A STEADY INCOME IS BETTER THAN A REPUTATION FOR BEING BRILLIANT. IT TAKES CONSIDERABLE KNOWLEDGE TO REALIZE THE EXTENT OF ONE'S IGNORANCE. GET YOUR FACTS FIRST, THEN YOU CAN DISTORT THEM AS YOU PLEASE. DON'T ARGUE, JUST EXPLAIN WHY YOU'RE RIGHT. ALWAYS REMEMBER THAT YOU'RE UNIQUE, JUST LIKE EVERYONE ELSE. I CAN RESIST EVERYTHING EXCEPT TEMPTATION.

Biofeedback Chart G

O NOBLE GUARDIAN OF MY HEART IN TWILIGHT'S HUSH, WHERE DREAMS AND SHADOWS BLEND, THY VISAGE SHINES, MY TRULY FAITHFUL FRIEND. WITH RUGGED GRACE THY FORM DOTH PROUDLY STAND, A BASTION FIRM, BOTH GENTLE AND YET GRAND. THINE EYES LIKE ORBS OF DEEPEST BLUE, REFLECT THE SKIES ~ ETERNAL, VAST, AND TRUE. THY BROW IS MARKED WITH WISDOM'S NOBLE TRACE, EACH LINE A TESTAMENT TO STRENGTH AND GRACE. WITH COURAGE SUBLIME, THOU MEETEST THE RISING SUN. A A WARRIOR FIERCE ~ YET KIND TO EVERYONE. THY VOICE, A MELODY SO RICH AND RARE, DOTH WEAVE A CHARM BEYOND COMPARE. O MAN OF VIRTUE, COURAGE, TRUTH, AND MIGHT, THY HUMBLE PRESENCE CASTS AWAY THE DARKEST NIGHT. WITH TENDER CARE, THY HANDS BOTH STRONG AND FAIR, LIFT ME HIGH AND BANISH MY DESPAIR. THY NOBLE ARMS, A FORTRESS AGAINST THE STORM OF LIFE'S FIERCE CRY, DO SHELTER ME BENEATH THE STARRY SKY. O GALLANT KNIGHT OF CHIVALROUS DEED, THY VIRTUE RADIANT AND BRIGHT, DOTH DOTH SET MY SOUL AFLAME WITH PASSIONATE DELIGHT. TO THEE, MY SOUL'S ETERNAL GUIDE, MY LOVE, MY FRIEND, MY JOY, MY PRIDE, WITH GRATITUDE MY HEART DOTH SING, O NOBLE GUARDIAN, MY EVERYTHING. THY COURAGE LIKE THE LION'S MIGHTY ROAR, DEFENDS THE WEAK, AND OPENS EVERY DOOR. IN TIMES OF TRIAL, THOU STANDEST PROUD AND TALL. THY HANDS, STRENGTHENED BY UNENDING TOIL, YET GENTLY TOUCH ~ IN LOVE'S SWEET TURMOIL. THEY CRADLE DREAMS AND BANISH SORROW'S FROWN, WITH EVERY TOUCH, THOU WEAREST LOVE'S BRIGHT CROWN. O NOBLE KNIGHT, MY GUARDIAN AND MY FRIEND, IN THEE, MY HEART SHALL EVERMORE DEPEND. FOR IN THY LOVE, I FIND MY TRUEST SELF. WITH THEE, MY SOUL IS FILLED WITH BOUNDLESS WEALTH. THY SPIRIT, NOBLE, VALIANT AND BOLD, A TALE OF HONOR, TIME AND AGAIN RETOLD. THY HEART, A TREASURE RARE AND PURE, OF LOVE UNYIELDING, STEADFAST AND SURE. WITH EVERY BREATH, IN AWE I STAND, A HUMBLE WITNESS TO THY GENTLE HAND. LOVE AND HONOR INTERTWINE, A PERFECT PORTRAIT OF THY SOUL DIVINE.

Biofeedback Chart H

IN THE LABYRINTH OF CITY LIGHTS I FOUND YOU ~ MY SERENE SERENADE. YOUR PRESENCE IS MY FAVORITE SONG ~ A MELODY THAT DANCES IN MY BLOOD, AWAKENING DREAMS LONG BURIED. YOUR LAUGHTER IS THE SUN BREAKING THROUGH THE STORM CLOUDS IN MY MIND, A BLISSFUL WARMTH THAT MELTS AWAY MY FEARS AND MAKES THE WORLD SEEM ALRIGHT AGAIN. TOGETHER, WE'RE WEAVING PRECIOUS MOMENTS INTO ETERNITY. EVERY WHISPERED SECRET, EVERY STOLEN GLANCE, IS A SACRED VOW SEALED IN THE LANGUAGE ONLY OUR HEARTS UNDERSTAND. OUR SOULS CONVERSE IN SILENCE, AND IN THE SPACES BETWEEN WORDS ~ WHERE LOVE SPEAKS THE LOUDEST, IN YOUR ARMS, I'VE FOUND MY TRUE HOME. YOU ARE THE CALM IN MY CHAOS, THE CERTAINTY IN MY MIND, THE BLESSED LOVE I THOUGHT I'D NEVER FIND. YOU ARE MY UNWRITTEN STORY, THE MUSE TO EVERY SONG UNSUNG. WITH YOU, THE MUNDANE BECOMES MAGICAL, EVERYDAY MOMENTS ETCHED INTO THE CANVAS OF MY HEART. YOU ARE THE REASON BEHIND MY SMILES, THE STRENGTH IN MY WEAK MOMENTS, MY PARTNER, MY LOVER, MY BEST FRIEND. IN YOUR SWEET EMBRACE, I FIND A SACRED SANCTUARY WHERE I CAN CAST ASIDE MY MASK AND TRULY BE MYSELF. YOU ARE MY HARBOR, MY REFUGE, THE ONE WHO TRULY SEES ME AND LOVES ME FOR ALL THAT I AM, AND ALL THAT I HOPE TO BE. EACH DAY WITH YOU IS A NEW CHAPTER, A STORY OF LOVE, RESILIENCE, AND HOPE. YOU INSPIRE ME TO DREAM BIGGER, REACH HIGHER, AND LOVE DEEPER. IN YOUR LOVE, I'VE FOUND MY ANCHOR, THE FORCE THAT KEEPS ME STEADY, EVEN WHEN LIFE'S WAVES THREATEN TO KNOCK ME DOWN. YOU ARE MY FOREVER, THE ONE I CHOOSE AGAIN AND AGAIN, IN THIS LIFE AND BEYOND. YOU'RE A PRECIOUS GIFT I CHERISH, A TREASURE I HOLD DEAR, A BEACON OF LIGHT IN A WORLD SO TREACHEROUS AND DARK. IN YOU, I'VE FOUND MY PERFECT IMPERFECT, A LOVE THAT'S REAL, SUBLIME, AND BEAUTIFUL. I VOW TO LOVE YOU TODAY, TOMORROW, AND ALWAYS, WITH ALL THAT I AM AND ALL THAT I HOPE TO BE. TOGETHER, WE ARE A FORCE OF NATURE, A SYMPHONY OF LOVE AND LIGHT THAT ASCENDS TO THE REALM OF THE DIVINE.

SECTION

4

THE
BOOSTER
EXERCISES

The Booster Exercises are an important supplement to the Power Exercises. Do the Booster Exercises two or three times a week, or more often if you're suffering from severe stress or eyestrain.

The Booster Exercises will reduce your stress level, relax your eyes, and improve the flow of nutrients in and around the eyes. These powerful exercises will quickly relieve headaches, eyestrain, and mental overload from reading or working at a computer.

Because the purpose of these exercises is to relieve stress, there's no time limit. They are so relaxing and refreshing that many people enjoy doing them for long periods of time. Do what works best for you. If you feel you only need to do them for a few minutes, that's fine too.

Booster Exercise #1: Hydrotherapy

What It Is: Hold a hot washcloth against your closed eyes.

What It Does: Stimulates the nutrient flow to your eyes, making them healthier and more attractive. Don't skip Hydrotherapy. It's a powerful technique that can reduce wrinkles and will make your eyes sparkle with new health and vitality!

How to Do It:

Step 1: Put a large bowl of really hot water on a table. The water should be as hot as you can comfortably stand it, but not so hot that it scalds your eyes.

Step 2: Dip a washcloth in the hot water and hold it against your closed eyes for about 10 seconds. Gently massage your closed eyes with the hot washcloth.

Dip the washcloth in the hot water again and repeat the procedure. Continue doing this for 10 minutes and repeat the affirmation "My eyes are getting better and my vision is improving!" When the hot water cools down, refill the bowl with more hot water.

An important variation is to have a bowl of ice-cold water next to the bowl of hot water. Alternate 10 seconds of hot water with 10 seconds of ice-cold water. Use a different washcloth for each bowl. This is very stimulating and will make your eyes tingle and feel wonderfully invigorated.

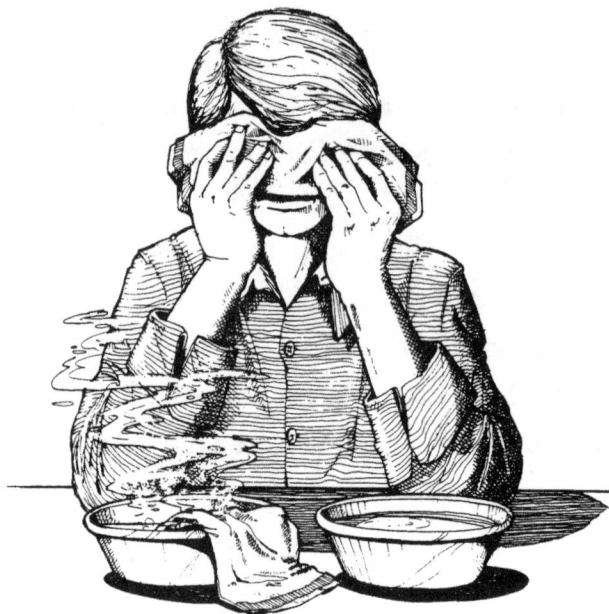

Booster Exercise #2: Palming

What It Is: Close your eyes and cover them with your cupped hands so that no light gets in. This exercise was devised by ophthalmologist William Bates and is an effective way of neutralizing eyestrain and nearpoint stress.

You can do it at a table, or in a comfortable chair, or lying down. Since the goal is relaxation, you may find it helpful to use cushions or pillows to support your arms so you are not straining to keep them in position.

Palming can also sharpen your vision—often dramatically. Many people enjoy doing it for up to 30 minutes as a form of meditation and stress relief. Try to keep your mind blank so that you're not worrying or thinking about your problems. This is your quiet time to relax and retreat into your inner space. An effective method of keeping your mind blank is to focus your attention on your breathing. Every time your mind wanders, bring it back to your breathing.

Instead of keeping your mind blank, you can visualize happy scenes or incidents in your life. Alternatively, you can pray, or repeat the affirmation, or listen to music. Make Palming a positive, enjoyable experience that you look forward to.

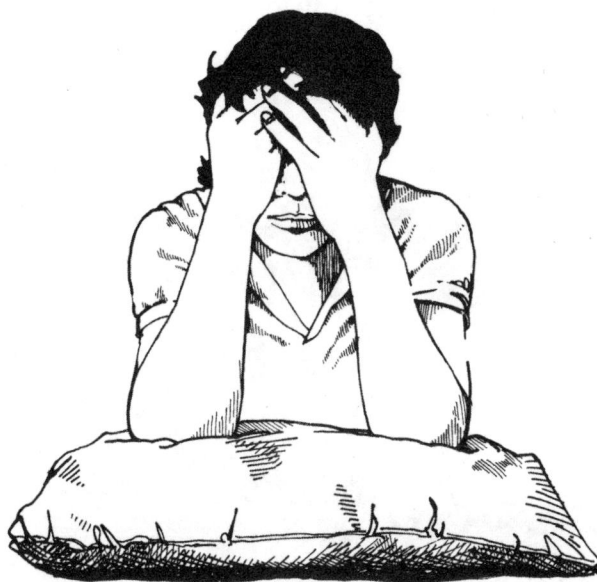

What It Does: Relieves visual stress and eyestrain. Improves nutrient flow and makes your eyes healthier. You will enjoy Palming. It's very pleasant and relaxing and will leave your eyes feeling energized and refreshed.

How to Do It:

Step 1: If you wear glasses, remove them. Close your eyes and cover them with cupped hands so no light gets in. Rest the base of your palms on your cheekbones and cross your hands on your forehead. Make sure that your hands, eyelids, and eyebrows are relaxed, and don't press on your eyes or your forehead.

Step 2: Breathe slowly and deeply and try to feel a sensation of warm, pulsating, healing energy in your eyes. Keep your mind blank, or focus your attention on your breathing, or repeat the affirmation "My eyes are getting better and my vision is improving!"

Booster Exercise #3: Light Therapy

What It Is: With your eyes closed, switch a bright light on and off in time to your breathing.

What It Does: Gives the iris sphincter muscle a good workout. Stimulates the flow of nutrients inside your eyes and makes them healthier.

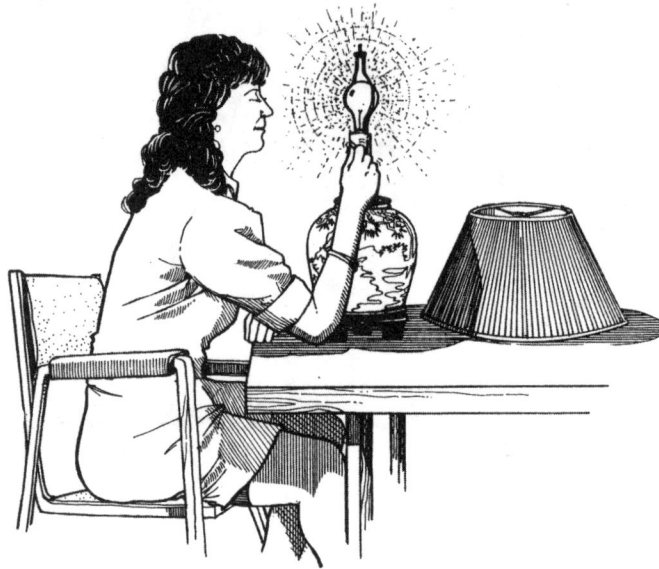

How to Do It:

Step 1: If you wear glasses, remove them. Sit about 12 inches in front of an unshaded 150-watt light, preferably incandescent, with your eyes closed and relaxed. If the light is too bright, move the lamp farther away; then reduce the distance as the light becomes more comfortable.

Step 2: Breathe slowly and deeply. As you inhale, switch the light on. As you exhale, switch it off. Concentrate on the sensation of warm, pulsating, healing energy in your eyes. Do this for up to 10 minutes. For best results, get an extension cord or surge protector with an on/off switch.

(inhale / on) > (exhale / off) > (inhale / on) > (exhale / off) > (inhale / on) > . . .

An important variation is to leave the light on. Don't switch it on and off. Just bathe your closed eyes in the bright light and slowly move your head from side to side. Concentrate on the sensation of warm, pulsating, healing energy in your eyes. Repeat the affirmation "My eyes are getting better and my vision is improving!"

Booster Exercise #4: Acupressure

What It Is: Massage the acupressure points around your eyes.

What It Does: Stimulates *chi energy* in your eyes, invigorating them and making them healthier. The acupressure techniques seem to exert a powerful healing effect. Some people report the sensation of rays of healing energy streaming out of the eyes! The exercises can also relieve eyestrain and headaches from too much reading or working at a computer.

How to Do It:

If you wear glasses, remove them. Firmly massage the acupressure points until they feel slightly sore without actually hurting. When doing the exercises, repeat the affirmation "My eyes are getting better and my vision is improving!"

Variation One

Step 1: Put your thumbs on the acupressure points shown in the diagram. For most people, the acupressure point is a small knob of bone that slightly protrudes inside the eye socket just below the eyebrow.

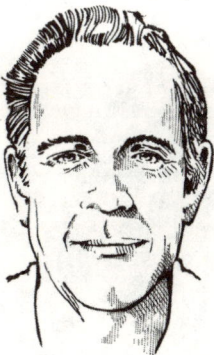

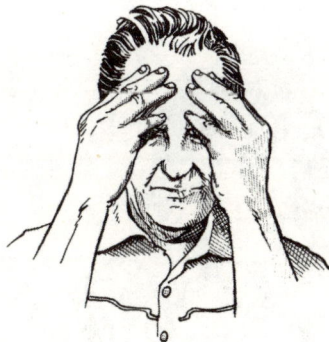

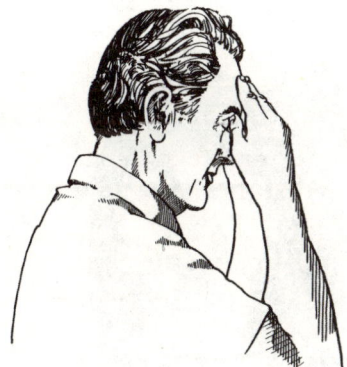

Step 2: Close your eyes and firmly press the acupressure points for about a second; then release for about a second. Continue to press and release for about a minute:

press > release > press > release > press > release > press > release > press > . . .

Variation Two

Step 1: Put your thumb and index finger of one hand on the acupressure points shown in the diagram. These are located on each side of the bridge of your nose.

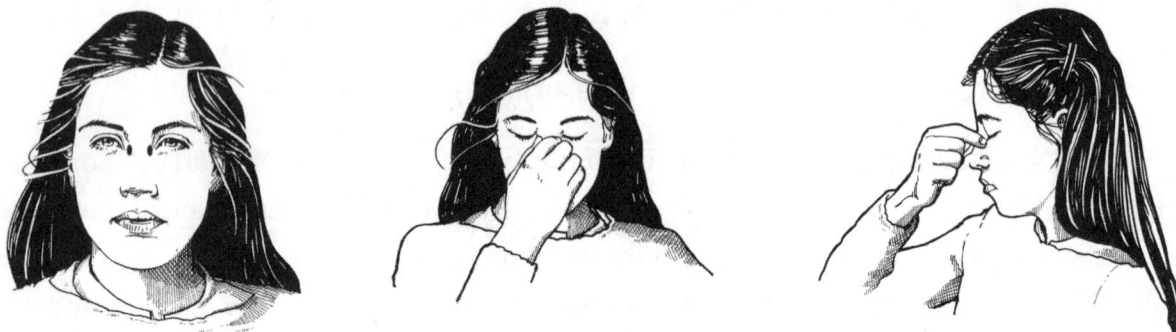

Step 2: Close your eyes and firmly massage the bridge of your nose between your eyes by squeezing for about a second, then releasing for about a second. Continue to squeeze and release for about a minute:

squeeze > release > squeeze > release > squeeze > release > squeeze > . . .

Variation Three

Step 1: Put one or two fingers on the acupressure points shown in the diagram, which are located on the crest of the cheekbones just below the eye sockets.

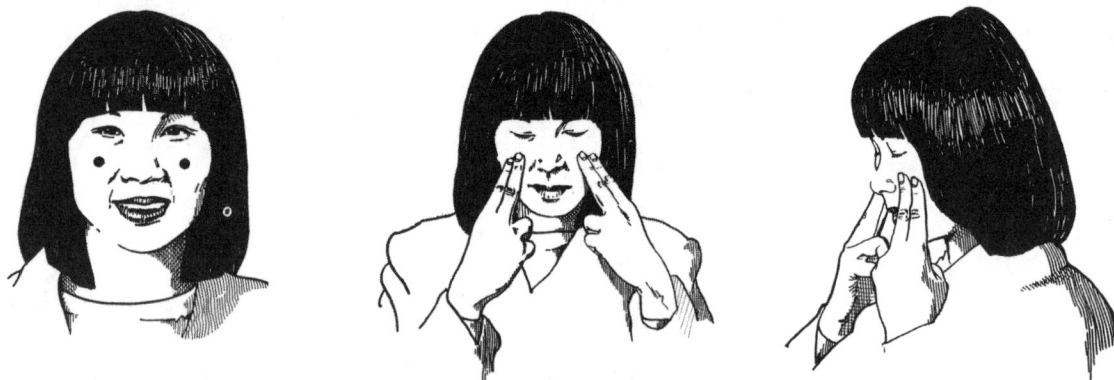

Step 2: Close your eyes and firmly massage the acupressure points by moving the skin in small circles. Change direction every few seconds.

Variation Four

Step 1: Put your thumbs in the pit of your temples. Now close your eyes and firmly stroke the upper and lower rims of your eye sockets from nose to temple. Use the section of your index fingers between the first and second joints.

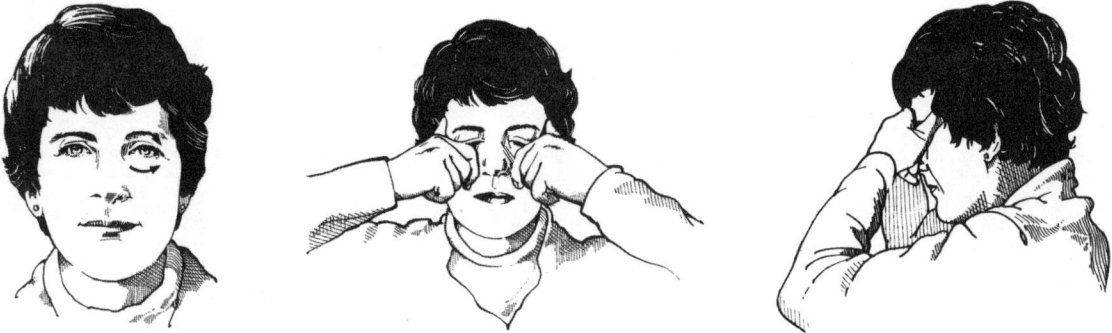

Step 2: Continue to alternately stroke the upper and lower rims of your eye sockets. You can use skin cream or mineral oil to avoid stretching the skin:

upper > lower > upper > lower > upper > lower > upper > lower > upper > ...

Variation Five

Step 1: When you've mastered all the previous variations, combine them into a stimulating massage of your entire eye region. Do a few seconds of Variation 1, then Variation 2, then Variation 3; then massage the entire rim of your eye sockets as in Variation 4. Go back and forth between the variations and give your entire eye region a really good acupressure massage.

Step 2: Instead of just massaging the acupressure points, we recommend that you increase the amount of stimulation by tapping the acupressure points and the entire eye region several times a second with the pads or tips of your fingers. Use two or three fingers for the most powerful effect.

tap > tap > tap > tap > tap > tap > tap > tap > tap > tap > tap > tap > tap > . . .

SECTION

5

THE
FUSION
EXERCISES

One of the goals of the Power Vision Program is to get rid of negative visual habits through a process known as *disembedding,* and replace them with positive new visual habits that help you see better and make your eyes healthier and more relaxed.

The Fusion Exercises are a powerful disembedding technique that improves the connection between accommodation and convergence, and will make your entire visual system more flexible and responsive. You should practice the exercises until you can do them easily. If you wear reading glasses or corrective lenses, you may need them for the exercises.

Make copies of the Fusion Charts so that you can hold them in your hand. In the beginning, the Fusion Exercises may cause some discomfort, in which case close your eyes and breathe slowly and deeply until the discomfort subsides; then resume the exercise. Don't overdo it. Stay within your comfort zone as much as possible. We recommend doing one exercise at a time. When you master it and can do it easily, go to the next exercise. Don't take on more than you can handle.

> **The Fusion Exercises will put you in a visual space you never knew existed!**

Although the Fusion Exercises may seem complicated, they are easy if you simply follow the directions step-by-step and don't give up. Don't get angry or frustrated! Even if it takes a while, just follow the directions and master the exercises one at a time. You will find them interesting—perhaps fascinating—because they will reveal part of your visual system that you were not aware of. They will put you in a visual space you never knew existed!

The Fusion Exercises are extremely important if you have presbyopia or hyperopia. They will make your inner lenses more flexible and increase your range of clear vision.

If you can't do any of them, you probably have an abnormally weak eye or a lazy eye and must fix that first using an eyepatch.

Fusion Warmup

Before doing the Fusion Exercises, you must be able to slightly cross your eyes.

How to Do It: Breathe slowly and deeply in front of a blank wall so you don't get distracting double images. As you inhale, cross your eyes by looking at the tip of your nose so that you see both sides of your nose at the same time. As you exhale, stop looking at the tip of your nose and uncross your eyes. Cross and uncross your eyes in time to your breathing until you can do it easily. Remember to blink every few seconds to keep your eyes lubricated.

(inhale / cross) > (exhale / uncross) > (inhale / cross)
> (exhale / uncross) > (inhale / cross) > . . .

If you can't do this, do Pushups (Power Exercise #4) and work at maintaining a single image as close to your nose as possible. Within a few days you should be able to cross your eyes and see both sides of the tip of your nose easily.

Alternatively, look at one side of the tip of your nose with one eye closed; then look at the other side of the tip of your nose with the other eye closed. Go back and forth from one eye to the other; then try to see both sides of the tip of your nose with both eyes open.

Fusion Exercise #1: Eccentric Circles

What It Does: Improves eye coordination, binocularity, and stereopsis—the ability to see in three dimensions.

How to Do It: Hold the circles at your usual reading distance and slowly cross your eyes. The sets of circles will fuse together to form a strong third set with a weaker set on each side. Now look at the central dot on the central set and hold it steady; then run your gaze around the inner circle.

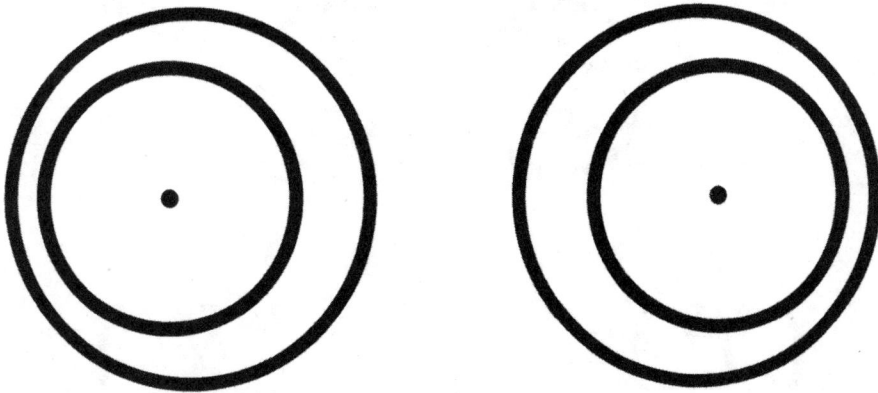

You will probably need to tilt your head slightly to get the images aligned. Breathe slowly and deeply and blink every few seconds to keep your eyes lubricated. The inner circle will suddenly rise above the outer circle to create an interesting three-dimensional effect. If you wear reading glasses or corrective lenses, you may need them for this exercise.

Fusion Exercise #2: Fusion Charts

What It Is: Look at an image on the Fusion Chart; then cross your eyes until you see a central image with a fainter image on either side.

What It Does: Stretches and conditions the extraocular muscles and increases the flexibility of the focusing system. Disembeds negative focusing patterns.

How to Do It: Hold Fusion Chart (A) where you can see it clearly and look at the top row of faces. Breathe slowly and deeply. Cross your eyes, then slowly uncross them. The faces will fuse together to form a strong, stable central face with a fainter face on either side. You will probably need to tilt your head slightly to bring the faces into alignment. Remember to blink every few seconds to keep your eyes lubricated. If you wear reading glasses or corrective lenses, you may need them for this exercise.

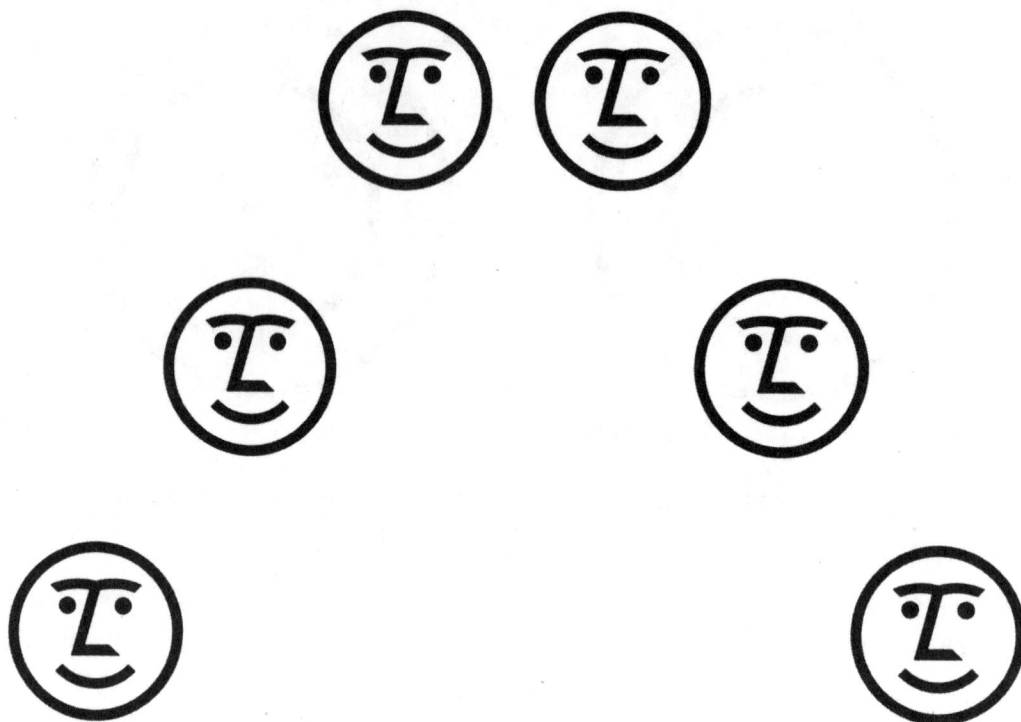

Fusion Chart (A)

Concentrate on the central face until it's completely solid and stable. The best way to do this is to slowly run your gaze along the lines of the nose or the mouth. Start this exercise with the top row of faces. If you get distracted by the lower rows of faces, cover them up.

Another way of doing this is to hold a pencil just below the top row of faces, midway between the Fusion Chart and your nose. Now look at the pencil, and you will see the faces come together to form a third face in the middle.

Do the exercise with the top row until you can easily get a strong, stable central fused face with a fainter face on either side. Then repeat the exercise with the middle row, then the bottom row.

Repeat the exercise until you're proficient at getting the central fused faces to form easily. Then go from the fused face in the top row to the fused face in the middle row, then to the fused face in the bottom row. Go back and forth between the fused faces in the different rows. Don't rush. Spend a couple of seconds looking at each fused face until it's strong and stable.

top > middle > bottom > middle > top > middle >
bottom > top > middle > bottom > top > . . .

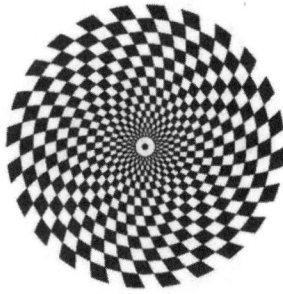

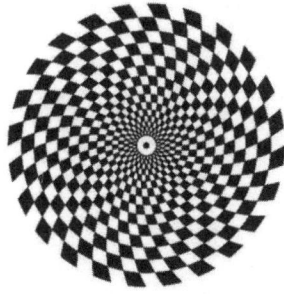

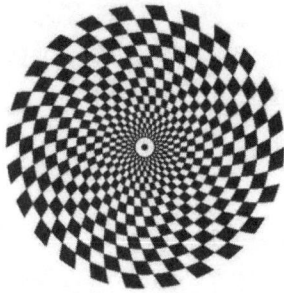

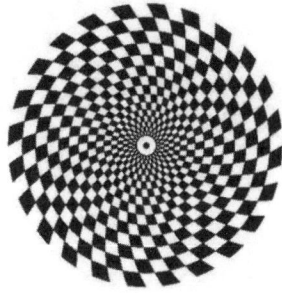

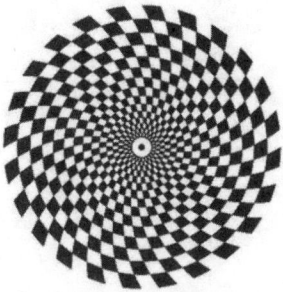

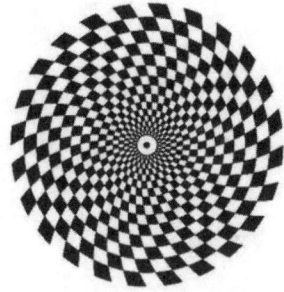

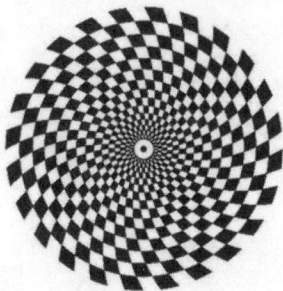

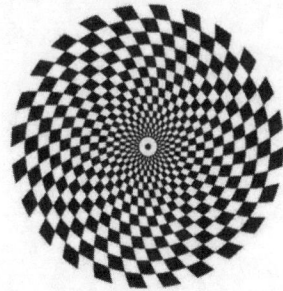

Fusion Chart (B)

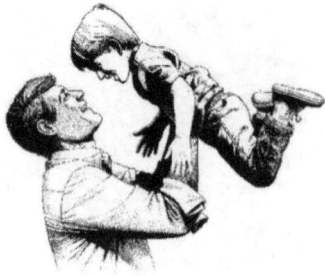

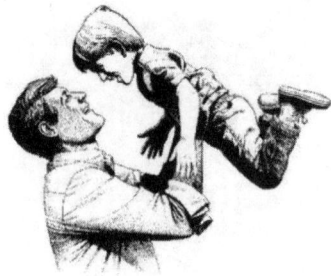

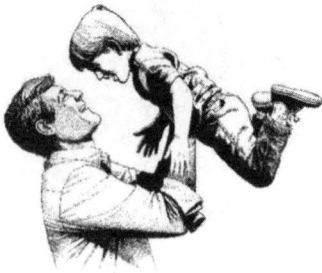

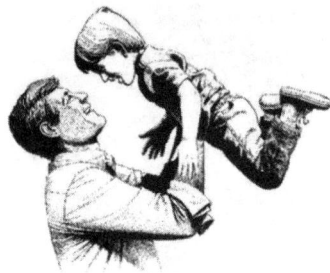

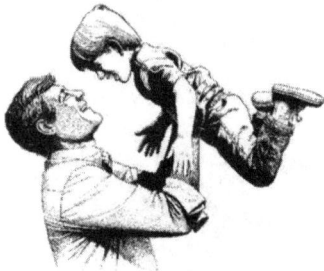

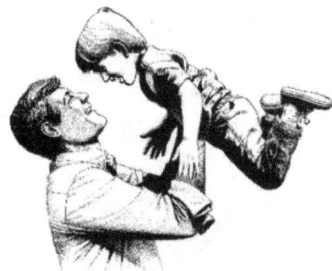

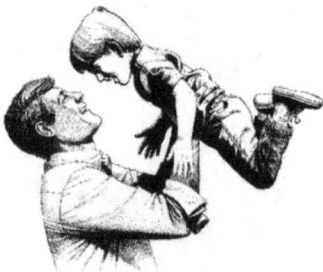

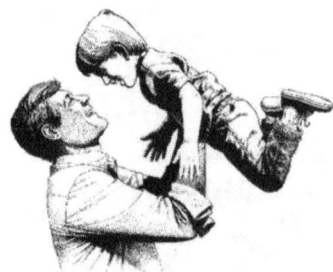

Fusion Chart (C)

DEMAND EXCELLENCE! BELIEVE IN YOURSELF AND ANYTHING IS POSSIBLE! GET THE KNOWLEDGE YOU NEED AND USE IT TO YOUR ADVANTAGE! LIVE! LOVE! LAUGH! LEARN TO BE BETTER THAN WHAT YOU ARE! THE SECRET OF GETTING AHEAD IS GETTING STARTED! BE ALL YOU CAN BE! EXCELLENCE IS NOT AN ACT BUT A HABIT! DO IT RIGHT! JUST DO IT! WINNERS MAKE IT HAPPEN! YOU HAVE THE POWER TO MAKE IT HAPPEN! BELIEVE IT AND ACHIEVE IT! LET'S MAKE THINGS BETTER! PLAN FOR SUCCESS! GOOD! BETTER! BEST! SUCCESS IS SWEET! PRACTICE WINNING EVERY DAY! REACH FOR THE STARS! TAKE ADVANTAGE OF THIS OPPORTUNITY! GOD HELPS THOSE WHO HELP THEMSELVES! YOU ARE A WINNER! ATTITUDE IS EVERYTHING! HOPE IS LIKE THE SUN! ENJOY IT! DEDICATION! BECAUSE YOU ARE WORTH IT! TRUST YOUR HIGHER POWER! YOU CAN DO IT! YES YOU CAN! PLAN TO SUCCEED! GET THE WINNING EDGE! DO IT NOW! GO CONFIDENTLY IN THE DIRECTION OF YOUR DREAMS! BELIEVE IT! DO IT! LIVE IT! DO WHATEVER IT TAKES! HIGH PERFORMANCE DELIVERY! THE BEST WAY TO MAKE YOUR DREAMS COME TRUE IS TO WAKE UP! HAVE FUN! ENJOY YOUR LIFE AND DANCE LIKE NOBODY'S WATCHING! AIM HIGH AND SUCCEED! FLY HIGH AND DARE TO DREAM! MAKE IT HAPPEN! REMEMBER, YOU HAVE THE STRENGTH, PATIENCE AND PASSION TO MAKE A DIFFERENCE IN YOUR LIFE!

Fusion Chart (D)

09•TWINKLE PRIVACY LAGOON VILLA ESTATE THERAPY HUG
10•GENUINE COMMAND PEACH SHOW COMFORT FOND
10•DIGNITY PARTNER THRIFT HARMONY PEARL FIT
11•ESTATE DEGREE ANTIQUE MANSION HUMOR
12•DEVELOP PRETTY CAVIAR PUPPY EXPLAIN
13•PERFUME ZOO CORDIAL RESPECT FAIR
14•PALACE HOLIDAY SHINE SNUGGLE
15•EMERALD PROTECT TOUCH HOLD
16•COMFORT RAPTURE TRUST JOY
17•ACTION MUSK CONFIDE HUGE
18•ETERNAL ADMIRE EMPATHY
19•BALLET SINCERE BED GIVE
20•REMEDY PURIFY SURVIVE
21•INSIGHT FUNDING VOW
22•EDUCATE HONEY GOLD
23•EXCITE BOLD PROVIDE
24•AWARD EXTRA REGAL
25•AMIABLE BELLE SUN
26•LISTEN GET SECURE
27•LOVE PEACE LORD
28•HEAVEN OVATION
29•NURSE WEALTHY
30•SERENE FLOWER
31•LOVING FAMILY
32•WORSHIP CHIC

09•TWINKLE PRIVACY LAGOON VILLA ESTATE THERAPY HUG
10•GENUINE COMMAND PEACH SHOW COMFORT FOND
10•DIGNITY PARTNER THRIFT HARMONY PEARL FIT
11•ESTATE DEGREE ANTIQUE MANSION HUMOR
12•DEVELOP PRETTY CAVIAR PUPPY EXPLAIN
13•PERFUME ZOO CORDIAL RESPECT FAIR
14•PALACE HOLIDAY SHINE SNUGGLE
15•EMERALD PROTECT TOUCH HOLD
16•COMFORT RAPTURE TRUST JOY
17•ACTION MUSK CONFIDE HUGE
18•ETERNAL ADMIRE EMPATHY
19•BALLET SINCERE BED GIVE
20•REMEDY PURIFY SURVIVE
21•INSIGHT FUNDING VOW
22•EDUCATE HONEY GOLD
23•EXCITE BOLD PROVIDE
24•AWARD EXTRA REGAL
25•AMIABLE BELLE SUN
26•LISTEN GET SECURE
27•LOVE PEACE LORD
28•HEAVEN OVATION
29•NURSE WEALTHY
30•SERENE FLOWER
31•LOVING FAMILY
32•WORSHIP CHIC

09•TWINKLE PRIVACY LAGOON VILLA ESTATE THERAPY HUG
10•GENUINE COMMAND PEACH SHOW COMFORT FOND
10•DIGNITY PARTNER THRIFT HARMONY PEARL FIT
11•ESTATE DEGREE ANTIQUE MANSION HUMOR
12•DEVELOP PRETTY CAVIAR PUPPY EXPLAIN
13•PERFUME ZOO CORDIAL RESPECT FAIR
14•PALACE HOLIDAY SHINE SNUGGLE
15•EMERALD PROTECT TOUCH HOLD
16•COMFORT RAPTURE TRUST JOY
17•ACTION MUSK CONFIDE HUGE
18•ETERNAL ADMIRE EMPATHY
19•BALLET SINCERE BED GIVE
20•REMEDY PURIFY SURVIVE
21•INSIGHT FUNDING VOW
22•EDUCATE HONEY GOLD
23•EXCITE BOLD PROVIDE
24•AWARD EXTRA REGAL
25•AMIABLE BELLE SUN
26•LISTEN GET SECURE
27•LOVE PEACE LORD
28•HEAVEN OVATION
29•NURSE WEALTHY
30•SERENE FLOWER
31•LOVING FAMILY
32•WORSHIP CHIC

09•TWINKLE PRIVACY LAGOON VILLA ESTATE THERAPY HUG
10•GENUINE COMMAND PEACH SHOW COMFORT FOND
10•DIGNITY PARTNER THRIFT HARMONY PEARL FIT
11•ESTATE DEGREE ANTIQUE MANSION HUMOR
12•DEVELOP PRETTY CAVIAR PUPPY EXPLAIN
13•PERFUME ZOO CORDIAL RESPECT FAIR
14•PALACE HOLIDAY SHINE SNUGGLE
15•EMERALD PROTECT TOUCH HOLD
16•COMFORT RAPTURE TRUST JOY
17•ACTION MUSK CONFIDE HUGE
18•ETERNAL ADMIRE EMPATHY
19•BALLET SINCERE BED GIVE
20•REMEDY PURIFY SURVIVE
21•INSIGHT FUNDING VOW
22•EDUCATE HONEY GOLD
23•EXCITE BOLD PROVIDE
24•AWARD EXTRA REGAL
25•AMIABLE BELLE SUN
26•LISTEN GET SECURE
27•LOVE PEACE LORD
28•HEAVEN OVATION
29•NURSE WEALTHY
30•SERENE FLOWER
31•LOVING FAMILY
32•WORSHIP CHIC

09•TWINKLE PRIVACY LAGOON VILLA ESTATE THERAPY HUG
10•GENUINE COMMAND PEACH SHOW COMFORT FOND
10•DIGNITY PARTNER THRIFT HARMONY PEARL FIT
11•ESTATE DEGREE ANTIQUE MANSION HUMOR
12•DEVELOP PRETTY CAVIAR PUPPY EXPLAIN
13•PERFUME ZOO CORDIAL RESPECT FAIR
14•PALACE HOLIDAY SHINE SNUGGLE
15•EMERALD PROTECT TOUCH HOLD
16•COMFORT RAPTURE TRUST JOY
17•ACTION MUSK CONFIDE HUGE
18•ETERNAL ADMIRE EMPATHY
19•BALLET SINCERE BED GIVE
20•REMEDY PURIFY SURVIVE
21•INSIGHT FUNDING VOW
22•EDUCATE HONEY GOLD
23•EXCITE BOLD PROVIDE
24•AWARD EXTRA REGAL
25•AMIABLE BELLE SUN
26•LISTEN GET SECURE
27•LOVE PEACE LORD
28•HEAVEN OVATION
29•NURSE WEALTHY
30•SERENE FLOWER
31•LOVING FAMILY
32•WORSHIP CHIC

09•TWINKLE PRIVACY LAGOON VILLA ESTATE THERAPY HUG
10•GENUINE COMMAND PEACH SHOW COMFORT FOND
10•DIGNITY PARTNER THRIFT HARMONY PEARL FIT
11•ESTATE DEGREE ANTIQUE MANSION HUMOR
12•DEVELOP PRETTY CAVIAR PUPPY EXPLAIN
13•PERFUME ZOO CORDIAL RESPECT FAIR
14•PALACE HOLIDAY SHINE SNUGGLE
15•EMERALD PROTECT TOUCH HOLD
16•COMFORT RAPTURE TRUST JOY
17•ACTION MUSK CONFIDE HUGE
18•ETERNAL ADMIRE EMPATHY
19•BALLET SINCERE BED GIVE
20•REMEDY PURIFY SURVIVE
21•INSIGHT FUNDING VOW
22•EDUCATE HONEY GOLD
23•EXCITE BOLD PROVIDE
24•AWARD EXTRA REGAL
25•AMIABLE BELLE SUN
26•LISTEN GET SECURE
27•LOVE PEACE LORD
28•HEAVEN OVATION
29•NURSE WEALTHY
30•SERENE FLOWER
31•LOVING FAMILY
32•WORSHIP CHIC

Fusion Chart (E)

Fusion Exercise #3: Fusion Flexing

What It Is: Use the fused central image for Flexing.

What It Does: Disembeds negative focusing patterns. Increases your focusing ability and improves your eye muscle coordination. Stimulates the nutrient flow inside your eyes and makes them healthier.

How to Do It: When you've mastered the Fusion Charts and can easily get a strong, stable fused image on the top row, use the fused image as the near object for Flexing (Power Exercise #2). Bring the chart as close to your eyes as possible before the fusion breaks up, then hold it steady at that distance with the fused image stable. Use any of the charts.

Breathe slowly and deeply. As you inhale, fuse the top row to form a stable central image. Then exhale and look at a far object such as a tree, automobile, person, building, or something across the room. Then look back at the fused central image.

Change focus in time to your breathing between the fused central image and the far object. When you can do this easily with the top row, do it using the fused central image on the other rows. Do the exercise with all the Fusion Charts. Blink every few seconds to keep your eyes lubricated.

If you experience any disorientation or discomfort, close your eyes and breathe slowly and deeply until you feel more relaxed; then resume the exercise. This is a powerful exercise that can improve the operation of your focusing system and increase your range of clear vision, so don't skip it.

(fused image) > (far object) > (fused image) > (far object) >
(fused image) > (far object) > . . .

Fusion Exercise #4: Fusion Pushups

What It Is: Use the fused central image for Pushups.

What It Does: Disembeds negative focusing patterns. Increases your focusing ability and improves your eye muscle coordination. Stimulates the nutrient flow inside your eyes and makes your eyes healthier.

How to Do It: When you've mastered the Fusion Charts and can easily get a stable fused image on the top row, use the fused image as the target for Pushups (Power Exercise #4). Use any of the Fusion Charts.

Breathe slowly and deeply and hold the chart at arm's length. Fuse the top row to form a stable central image; then inhale and bring the chart toward you as if you are doing a Pushup. Keep the fused image stable as you do this. Get as close to your eyes as possible before the fusion breaks up.

As you exhale, move the chart to arm's length. Go back and forth in time to your breathing with the central image fused and stable at all times. When you can do this easily with the top row, do it with the other rows. Blink frequently to keep your eyes lubricated.

(inhale / toward) > (exhale / away) > (inhale / toward) > (exhale / away) > . . .

When you can do this easily with the top row, do it with the other rows and with the other charts.

This is a powerful exercise that can improve the operation of your focusing system and increase your range of clear vision, so don't skip it. If you experience any disorientation or discomfort, close your eyes and breathe slowly and deeply until you feel more relaxed; then resume the exercise.

Fusion Exercise #5: Thumb Fusion

What It Is: Form a central fused image of your thumbs.

What It Does: Disembeds negative focusing patterns.

How to Do It: Make two fists with your thumbs up. Then hold them together at arm's length with the thumbs touching each other. Now fuse the thumbs. You will see a fused central thumb with a fainter thumb on either side of it.

Now slowly move your fists apart. Keep the central thumb fused and see how far you can go without losing fusion. Use a blank wall to avoid double images of objects in the background.

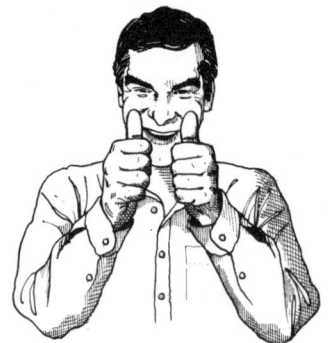

SECTION

6

THE
VISION
THERAPY
BREAK
THROUGH

Although vision therapy is usually considered to be a modern method of treating bad eyesight, it has its roots in the distant past. The Power Vision Program is a combination of procedures from many different disciplines, most of which have been tested in clinical practice and proved effective against a wide range of common visual problems.

Vision therapy originated more than 2,000 years ago, when the Indian spiritual master Pantanjali laid down the principles of yoga in his treatise *The Yoga Sutras*. Over the years, this great work has influenced the lives of millions of people and contains several important techniques for improving vision.

In addition to a total system of health care, Patanjali formulated exercises that cleanse the eyes, improve the performance of the extraocular muscles, and reduce stress by regulating breathing.

Yoga rapidly spread throughout Asia and produced a rich tradition of sacred knowledge and wisdom that endures to the present day. Pantanjali's followers developed eyecharts known as *yantras*, which improve eye coordination and saccadic eye movements.

This yantra was created by Tibetan monks. Simply run your gaze along the edge of the yantra all the way around, going into all the nooks and crannies. You can also use the yantra for Detailing (Power Exercise #6), in which case put it where it's slightly blurred.

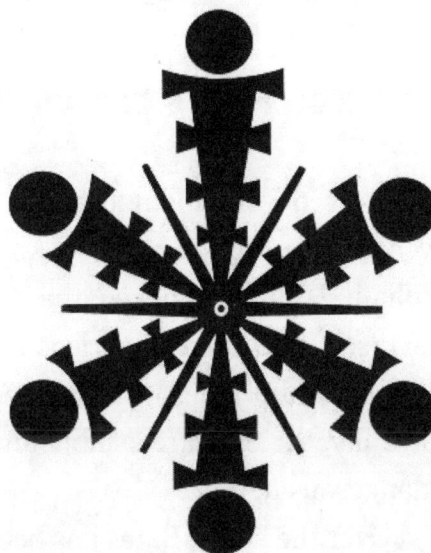

Early Treatment of Strabismus

The next advance came in the seventh century, when the Greek physician Paulus Aeginta treated strabismus (crossed eyes) using a mask with special eye holes. These forced the inward-turning eye to move out. Although the treatment sounds crude, it was widely used until the eighteenth century.

Further advances came in 1743 when the French scientist Leclerc realized that the inward turning eye was *lazy* and recommended covering the good eye in order to make the lazy eye work harder. This technique was improved in 1778 by the English physician Erasmus Darwin, who developed eye exercises to make the procedure more effective.

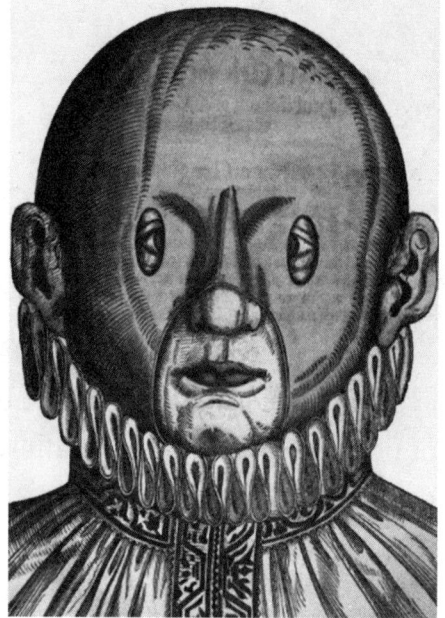

Bates: Heretic or Hero?

The next development came in the early part of the twentieth century, when the American ophthalmologist William H. Bates rocked the medical profession with his discoveries and theories. Although many patients acclaimed him a hero who helped restore their eyesight naturally, the eye care establishment condemned him as a dangerous heretic.

Over the years, Bates has been the subject of intense controversy, and the true value of his work has never been formally recognized. Bates attained a widespread following, and many books have been written about his theories and techniques. Regrettably, the eye care establishment has never seriously investigated his work and has consistently refused to publish anything supporting his method of improving vision.

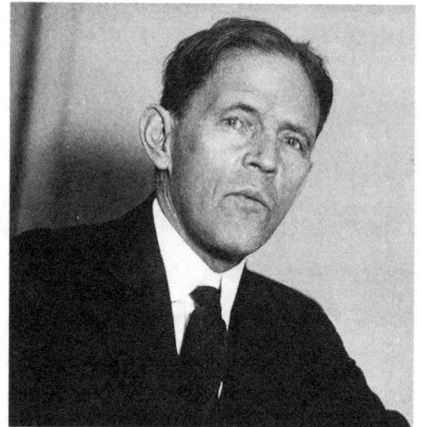

Disturbing Observations

Bates was born in 1860 in Newark, New Jersey. He graduated from Cornell University in 1881 and received his medical degree in 1885 from the College of Physicians and Surgeons. After serving as an attending physician at the Manhattan Eye and Ear Hospital, Bellevue Hospital, and the New York Eye Infirmary, he taught ophthalmology at the New York Postgraduate Medical School from 1886 to 1891.

As a result of examining thousands of patients every year, Bates became increasingly disturbed over the fact that what he observed often contradicted what he had been taught and was teaching his students.

Bates then began to explore the concept that vision could be improved naturally through exercise instead of corrective lenses. In 1891, he published an article in a medical journal on eliminating nearsightedness by this means. He commented:

> "The theory that poor eyesight is incurable does not fit the observed facts. I have seen many cases in which errors of refraction recover spontaneously or change their form. It has long been the custom of ophthalmologists to ignore these troublesome facts or try to explain them away."

Thirty Years of Research

During the next 30 years, Bates continued his research and in 1921 published a book called *Perfect Sight Without Glasses*. In this book, he claimed that visual problems are caused by stress. He outlined a system for exercising and relaxing the visual system—the Bates method—and claimed that it could cure astigmatism, myopia, hyperopia, presbyopia, glaucoma, and cataracts.

During this period, Bates was in private practice in New York, where he helped numerous patients improve their vision with his method. As news of his success became widely known, patients flocked to his office, some of whom became disciples. He trained them as practitioners and set up vision improvement centers in several different cities.

Persecution and Prosecution

Although Bates submitted the results of his investigations to medical journals, instead of stimulating further research, his findings were ridiculed and condemned. Bates pleaded with his former colleagues to carry out an investigation. They refused, and he soon found himself isolated and ignored.

As the new method of vision care began to spread, the medical establishment attacked him. In 1928 he was expelled from the American Medical Association, which filed a civil lawsuit against him in 1929, charging him with unlawfully advertising a medical practice. After a two-year legal battle that went all the way to the Supreme Court, Bates was acquitted. Victorious but with his health ruined, he died a few months later at the age of 71.

It's important to note that the subject of the lawsuit was unlawful advertising—not fraud. Furthermore, all medical practices that advertise their services, including clinics, treatment centers, and hospitals, rely on the Bates case as legal precedent. Hence, in a bizarre twist of fate that the eye care establishment will never accept, Bates can be rightfully considered as one of the founding fathers of modern medicine!

Celebrity Endorsements

Following Bates's death, his disciples continued to popularize the method, and books and newspaper articles were published on the subject. The Bates method became something of a craze. Popular interest was reflected in a movie starring Joan Bennet and Franchot Tone, where the hero got rid of his glasses by exercising his eyes.

Several authors, including E. A. van Vogt and the famous novelist Aldous Huxley, improved their eyesight using the Bates method. Huxley's case is especially significant because he was severely myopic and on the edge of blindness before beginning the treatment. As he reported:

"My vision was steadily getting worse. Even with greatly strengthened glasses, I could hardly see anything at all. A friend told me about the Bates method and I decided to try it. The results were astonishing. Within a couple of months I was reading without glasses.

Better still, the chronic tensions and headaches which had troubled me for years cleared up completely. My case is not unique. Thousands of other people have used this method with success."

The Trial of Margaret Corbett

Under the new leadership of Dr. Harold Peppard and Margaret Darst Corbett, the number of Bates method practitioners steadily increased. Vision improvement centers were set up throughout the United States and in other countries. Large numbers of people discarded corrective lenses or avoided them in the first place.

Alarmed by the growing popularity of the Bates method, the eye care establishment attacked Corbett and brought her to trial on the grounds that she was practicing optometry without a license. Like Bates, she was charged with a simple procedural violation, not fraud.

Corbett responded by filling the courtroom with more than 500 witnesses, many of whom testified how the Bates method had improved their eyesight. Some of the witnesses were movie stars and the trial was widely publicized. One witness reported that he had been almost blind from cataracts, but after treatment could read for eight hours at a stretch without glasses.

Snowstorm of Public Protest

Optometrists and ophthalmologists all over the United States anxiously awaited the verdict. In January 1941, the court found Corbett not guilty. Dismayed by her victory, the eye care establishment then introduced a bill into the California State Legislature making it unlawful for anyone to teach any method of exercising or relaxing the eyes without a medical or optometric license.

Corbett responded with a radio broadcast in which she urged the public to ask their elected representatives to vote against it. She attacked the *medical monopoly* and *eyeglass racket*, which she claimed were keeping the public enslaved to optical products.

Corbett's campaign succeeded. A snowstorm of letters opposing the bill descended on the legislators. The bill was defeated, and eight senators who had regularly supported measures favored by the medical establishment in the past voted against it. Other legal victories were also recorded for the Bates movement. In 1951, Clara Hackett was acquitted by a grand jury in New York on a similar charge.

Success in the War Effort

During the Second World War, thousands of young men used the Bates method to improve their vision so they could pass military eye examinations. After the war, the Veteran's Administration approved the Bates method for rehabilitation work with returning veterans.

Corbett died in 1961. Lacking a leader, the Bates movement lost a lot of momentum. During the last few decades, however, there's been a resurgence of interest. Several new books have been published on the subject and members of the public continue to report getting good results, but the eye care establishment continues to downplay the method.

The Helmholtz Theory of Accommodation

The eye's ability to change focus puzzled scientists and physicians for more than 400 years. In fact, it was only in the middle of the nineteenth century that the German scientist Hermann von Helmholtz published the results of his famous investigations, in which he claimed that the eye changes focus by changing the shape of the inner lens.

The Helmholtz theory forms the basis of modern eye care and is universally accepted by the eye care profession. Bates disputed this theory, stating that the inner lens is not a factor. Instead, he claimed that the extraocular muscles focus the eye by squeezing the eyeball and changing its length.

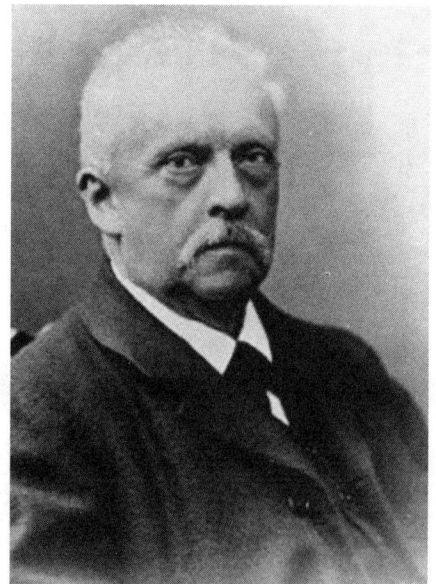

Flaws in the Helmholtz Theory

Although the Helmholtz theory provides a satisfactory explanation for most clinical observations, there are some curious phenomena that it fails to account for:

- Atropine is a drug that paralyzes the ciliary muscle and prevents it from changing the shape of the inner lens. In some cases, however, patients are still able to change focus.

- A similar phenomenon was also observed in cataract surgery in the nineteenth century, when the inner lens was simply removed. At that time, replacement lenses had not been invented. According to the Helmholtz theory, there should be no accommodation, but in many cases the patient could still change focus.

- Bates observed that in some conditions such as astigmatism, the refractive error and shape of the eyeball could spontaneously change.

Bates was disturbed by these phenomena and found that although most ophthalmologists had accepted the Helmholtz theory without question, Helmholtz had stated that his results were inconclusive. As ophthalmologist Tscherning pointed out:

"The disciples of Helmholtz proclaimed as truth what the master only deemed as probable."

Why Bates Became a Heretic

To his credit, Bates patiently duplicated Helmholtz's experiments for four years and tried to resolve the matter. Whereas Helmholtz merely relied on observation, Bates tried to obtain solid evidence by photographing the movement of the inner lens. Like Helmholtz, he was unable to get conclusive results.

Bates then experimented with animals and fish, and found that in some cases the extraocular muscles are indeed responsible for accommodation. Bates concluded that the same mechanism must take place in the human eyes. Unfortunately for Bates, science proved him wrong.

Although Bates's disciples claimed that he developed a new theory, the idea that the eyeball changes its shape is an old theory that was held by Listing, Sturm, and other scientists in the early nineteenth century. However, they abandoned the theory when Helmholtz published his results.

The Mystery Remains Unsolved

Although Bates has been criticized for his experimental methods, he must be given credit for attempting to replicate Helmholtz's results. It was another 50 years before researchers finally obtained conclusive evidence supporting the Helmholtz theory. In 1940, thanks to developments in infrared photography, the changes in the inner lens were finally recorded on film.

In fairness to Bates, the anomalous effects of atropine and cataract surgery have been well documented by other researchers. However, neither Bates's theory nor the Helmholtz theory accounts for the phenomena, and a satisfactory explanation has never been proposed.

It should be noted that Bates developed his method when not much was known about the structure of the eye or the way the visual system works. He was a pioneer, and like many pioneers, he made mistakes. He relied on an obsolete theory to explain his results, and he probably made too many claims, leaving himself open to attack by his critics.

> **Bates developed his method when not much was known about the structure of the eye or the way the visual system works.**

Why the Establishment Rejected Bates

Doctors do not find it easy to give up a theory upon which they have based their work for years. Not only do they demand proof of the new theory, but they often display antagonism, as though the new theory is an attempt to undermine their position. This is especially true of traditional optometrists, who derive most of their income from prescribing and selling corrective lenses and have no interest in natural methods of vision improvement.

However, in fairness to Bates's critics, we agree that some of his ideas and claims seem to be unbelievable. Nevertheless, if one actually reads his book and understands his procedures, the impression is that Bates was a sincere and conscientious investigator.

Principles of the Bates Method

Bates believed that poor vision is caused by stress and tension, which impair the performance of the extraocular muscles and distort the shape of the eyeball. He emphasized the importance of past experience, memory, and imagination as functions of the visual process. He also asserted that vision takes place in the brain, where it is coupled with memory and imagination, and that a stressful environment causes the visual system to malfunction.

According to Bates, relaxation is the key factor in improving vision. Covering the eyes and swinging the body are important parts of his method. He also advocated running the gaze along the edges of objects and the use of fine print as an aid to improving acuity.

Bates's disciples added more techniques to the method: Corbett emphasized blinking and changing focus between near and far; Peppard suggested using weaker glasses; Hauser pointed out the importance of nutrition; Huxley added the yoga technique of deep breathing; Kelley and Scholl developed new exercises based on psychotherapy.

Does the Bates Method Really Work?

Although many books have been written by his disciples and former patients who got good results, almost nothing has been published in the major eye care journals on the subject. In view of the widespread interest that the Bates method has inspired for over a century, we found this surprising when we began our own investigation a few years ago.

Bates claimed that his method could cure most common visual problems. Although the eye care establishment relentlessly attacked him, they failed to produce a shred of evidence that his claims were fraudlent. Instead, they resorted to fearmongering and slander, ridiculing the exercises as a dangerous waste of time.

It appears that Bates had data supporting his work but stated that it was "difficult to get this sort of thing published." Did this mean that he had carried out clinical studies but was censored by the major journals because of his unorthodox theories and methods? We may never know, but the fact remains that after his book was published, Bates was completely ostracized by the eye care establishment.

Nevertheless, Bates found friends among the intellectuals of that period. In 1944, ophthalmologist Walter Lancaster concluded:

"If one studies the Bates method with an open mind, one will be forced to admit that there are sound and fruitful ideas. With a more skillful technique, based on a wiser and more rational theory, the results will be even more impressive.

There is abundant evidence for the general proposition that exercises, repetition, practice, and learning lead to better performance and to the acquisition of skill. Many ocular conditions exemplify this principle."

Answers to Some Important Questions

Ophthalmologist Judd Beach agreed:

"It is customary to ridicule these sight training exercises as a waste of time. Patients who achieve improved vision do not agree. They are delighted to be able to discard their glasses in a number of common situations like recognizing friends on the street and reading signs.

One patient pointed out that it is useful to be able to sail without having to wipe spray off glasses, and it might be lifesaving to be able to recognize landmarks if his glasses blew off. Such advantages are too real to be laughed at."

Critics charged that the Bates method merely trains people to recognize blurred images without producing a real increase in acuity. Beach responded:

"If we could find out what makes these cases tick, we might get an answer to some important questions. These people are smart enough to know when they see vividly. They know that they are not getting a method of distinguishing blurred images—and they are discounting statements made by various ophthalmologists whom they feel should be stuffed and put in museums."

Mystery of the Clear Flashes

The *flashes* of clear vision are one of the most intriguing phenomena produced by the Bates method. Corbett explained:

> "For some people, improvement is a gradual sharpening of acuity. But for many, there are flashes of perfectly clear vision. As the patient progresses, the flashes become longer and more frequent, eventually blending into permanent better sight."

Bates incorrectly theorized that the eyeball changes shape during a clear flash. Some researchers now believe that a biofeedback effect may lower the pressure inside the eyeball and modify the focusing power of the lens. Other researchers suggest that tear fluid may form a natural contact lens, or that the brain can learn how to enhance a blurred image like a computer.

In 1947, optometrist James Gregg studied clear flashes under clinical conditions. One subject improved from 20/600 to 20/50. Another went from 20/200 to 20/20. However, he was unable to observe any changes in the structure of the eye. The following year, Beach reported:

> "Patients describe periods of intensely vivid vision, sometimes with 20/10 acuity. They are impatient with ophthalmologists for neglecting this experience. The keenness of vision may occur in one eye and later shift to the other. Or it may take place in both eyes at the same time."

In 1952, optometrist Elwin Marg studied the phenomenon under clinical conditions and confirmed that it was real, although neither the Bates theory nor the Helmholtz theory could explain it.

Typically, subjects improved their acuity from 20/300 to 20/50. Marg agreed with Bates that the phenomenon seemed similar to the accommodation observed in lens-less eyes resulting from cataract surgery. Like Gregg, Marg was unable to observe any changes in the shape of the eye.

That same year, French ophthalmologist Yves Le Grand confirmed Marg's findings and concluded that *negative accommodation* was the factor responsible for the effect.

Investigations of a Psychologist

In 1962, psychologist Charles Kelley published a remarkable paper confirming the effectiveness of the Bates method. Kelley's work is significant because he became a certified Bates practitioner in order to study the method firsthand. Kelley reported:

> "It was found that large improvements in acuity do occur as a consequence of Bates training, for example from 20/200 to 20/40. Furthermore, flashes of normal or greatly improved acuity lasting from a few seconds to several hours are induced by the methods. The frequency, duration, and vividness of these flashes are extended systematically by the Bates method.
>
> These flashes are not produced by tricks such as squinting or applying pressure to the eyeball. They appear to reflect refractive changes. Most people who persevere with the training are substantially improved, and many require weaker glasses or are able to dispense with glasses altogether."

The Evidence Piles Up

In 1968 optometrist V. L. Copeland reported flashes of improved acuity resulting from deep hypnotic relaxation. One patient showed an improvement from 20/700 to 20/40! These findings were later confirmed by Graham and Liebowitz, Lanyon and Giddings, Tobias, and Kaplan.

And in 1978, optometrist Philip Smith carried out a clinical study of the Bates method. Thirty-three out of thirty-four patients sharpened their acuity. Improvements ranged from 16% to 500%. Smith reported:

> "The patients consisted of presbyopes, hyperopes, and myopes. Following training, all became independent of their glasses to some extent. Eleven needed glasses only for reading or driving. The rest did not need them at all.
>
> All the patients experienced flashes of clear vision, with some able to maintain it constantly. Freedom from glasses was like music to their ears. The improvements in acuity represent a change in magnitude that cannot be ascribed merely to the interpretation of blurred images."

In addition to the clinical studies, many eye doctors have accumulated data throughout the years from patients who used the Bates method successfully, but have not published it. Because they don't know how to write a scientific paper, or don't want to risk being attacked by the eye care establishment, a lot of important information lies buried in their files.

The Establishment Opens Its Doors

In 1982, the *Journal of Optometric Vision Development*, which is devoted to behavioral optometry, published a detailed analysis of the Bates method by optometric scientist Raymond Gottlieb. The importance of this paper can be judged by the fact that the entire issue of the journal was devoted to it. Gottlieb reported:

> "After personal investigation of the Bates method led to the elimination of my own nearsightedness, I became convinced of the positive aspects of his system. Since that time, I have worked with patients and have achieved moderate success with the method.
>
> On the basis of personal experiences and an intuitive sense of the essential correctness of his ideas, I researched Bates' concepts and found that his work is important. Vision specialists should be aware of its possible utility in preventing and correcting nearsightedness."

Gottlieb went on to explain how Bates made some important observations about the factors leading to myopia, revealing a holistic approach that was surprisingly contemporary in its tone and content. Gottlieb concluded:

> "That Bates has been so maligned and misunderstood is a gross injustice which has impeded our investigation of important problems in vision care. It is clearly indicated that the work of Bates, so long ignored by the clinical communities, needs to be reexamined in an openminded scientific manner."

Where Bates's Critics Blundered

The Bates method has been frequently criticized. In particular, ophthalmologist Sorsby and optometrist Pollack analyzed Bates's theories, carefully pointing out the flaws. However, these critics made the serious error of trying to deny the evidence, the clinical observations, and the stream of positive reports from people who used the method. As Lancaster explained:

"They make the mistake of arguing that because Bates's theory of accommodation is incorrect, his whole method is unsound. The history of medicine is a long list of tentative theories later proved to be erroneous, but the facts they tried to explain remain firmly established, though the theories themselves are swept away. For example, quinine cured malaria and continued to cure it, though the theories invented to account for its action were wrong."

Huxley's rebuttal was also sharp and to the point:

"Sorsby entirely fails to distinguish between two different things: the evidence confirming the existence of the phenomenon and the theory advanced to explain the evidence. The phenomena of the Bates method are the marked improvements in vision which follow the practice of the techniques. The evidence for the occurrence of these phenomena can be supplied by thousands of persons who, like myself, have derived benefit from the method, and from the scores of trained instructors who teach it.

If Sorsby really wanted to know about the evidence, he would get in touch with reliable teachers of the method, watch them at work, and if his own vision is defective, try the method himself."

Bates's Theories Partly Confirmed

Although Bates made a mistake by insisting that the inner lens plays no part in accommodation, his ideas regarding the role of the extraocular muscles have been partly confirmed. Optometrist Stephen Miller, chairman of the Primary Care Division of the American Optometric Association, noted:

> "There has been some concern that when we focus, the pressure exerted on the eyeball puts stress on the external surface of the eye, which could cause myopia to increase."

Other evidence suggests that the extraocular muscles can deform the eyeball over a period of time. As Bates observed, astigmatism often varies considerably, worsening or reversing during periods of stress, then easing off when life returns to normal.

As a result of this phenomenon and similar evidence, many researchers now believe that although the extraocular muscles do not play a role in accommodation, they can deform the eyeball over a period of time. As Bates suggested, this may be a major factor in many common visual problems.

The Verdict on Bates

Nobel laureate Linus Pauling was once asked how he managed to generate so many good ideas. He replied that the secret was to generate lots of ideas, then get rid of the bad ones. Like Pauling, Bates had lots of ideas. However, he failed to eliminate all the bad ones. As a result, Bates's work contains inaccuracies and mistakes.

As previously discussed, critics suggest that the Bates method merely teaches the patient how to interpret blurred images. However, clinical investigations and numerous reports from patients confirm that a genuine improvement in acuity takes place, and in many cases the eyeball does in fact gradually change shape.

To clear up the mystery of the clear flashes, we analyzed the Bates method in light of modern advances in vision research and concluded that there are nine different mechanisms that can cause improved acuity, including the clear flashes. We explain these mechanisms at the end of Section 9.

The evidence shows that most of Bates's claims and concepts are in fact correct. However, his theory of accommodation is deeply flawed.

On balance, we believe that Bates made a significant contribution to visual science and should be given the recognition he deserves. All the published reports show that the Bates method is quite effective in improving acuity. Although it does not usually cure the underlying visual problem, it can often prevent it in the first place.

We must never forget that Bates was a pioneer who carried out investigations when the anatomy and functionality of the eyes were not well understood. We feel the time has come for the eye care establishment to reevaluate his work in a calm, objective, scientific manner instead of the hysterical fearmongering that has characterized so much of the criticism in the past.

Yes, his theory of accommodation was wrong. But there is an abundance of clinical and scientific evidence that most of his observations and theories were correct. Specifically:

- Vision takes place in the brain.

- Deep relaxation can improve acuity.

- Aphakic eyes can show accommodation.

- The adult visual system is not immutable.

- Vision can be improved through eye exercises.

- Stress causes the visual system to malfunction.

- Astigmatism can vary in its axis and magnitude.

- Edge discrimination training can improve acuity.

- Corrective lenses often aggravate visual problems.

- Eyes treated with atropine can show accommodation.

These observations are not trivial and form the foundation upon which much of behavioral optometry is based, although Bates has not been given any credit by any of the behavioral optometric organizations. It is time to correct that injustice. As Peppard concluded:

"The Bates method is controversial only to eye care professionals who do not use it. To those of us who do, the effectiveness of this technique is established beyond question."

Optometry: Birth of a Profession

In addition to Bates, many other eye care professionals made significant contributions to vision therapy. To appreciate the importance of their discoveries, however, we must view them in a historical context.

Corrective lenses date back to 1286, when the medieval scholar Francis Bacon discovered that a magnifying lens improved his ability to read manuscripts. A few years later, the Italian craftsmen Alexander de Spina and Salvino D'Armati attached small magnifying lenses to metal frames, and the first spectacles were born.

Long before the advent of the eye examination, spectacles were sold in marketplaces by jewelers, tinkers, and tailors. Vendors offered a selection that customers could try on and choose from. The spectacle trade rapidly spread throughout Europe and proved a blessing to many people.

Over the next few centuries, various types of lenses were developed to compensate for different visual problems, and the art of making and fitting spectacles was passed down from master to apprentice. Many spectacle makers set up proprietory schools where anyone could learn the trade and obtain a diploma.

The end of the nineteenth century saw the birth of optometry. Advances in optical science allowed spectacle vendors to perform basic eye examinations, and a new class of practitioners emerged who called themselves *refracting opticians*. Their techniques made spectacle selection more precise, and they decided to form a new profession.

Working hand-in-glove with the optical glass industry, refracting opticians founded the American Optometric Association in 1904, coining the term *doctor of optometry* to describe themselves. To standardize procedures, the apprenticeship system was abandoned and the proprietary schools were shut down.

Regulatory laws were passed and courses were set up in colleges and universities, teaching optometrists and ophthalmologists how to prescribe corrective lenses and diagnose eye diseases.

> **Long before the advent of eye examinations, spectacles were sold by jewelers, tinkers, and tailors.**

The Facade of Professional Unity

During the next few decades, intense legal conflicts took place in every state as the American Optometric Association battled the American Medical Association over treatment procedures and financial territory. These conflicts continue to the present day, with many eye doctors competing for patients and health care dollars.

The eye care establishment tries to downplay these conflicts and wants the public to think that eye doctors are a big happy family. That is misleading. Bitter rivalry between the different factions has seriously impeded the flow of information regarding major advances in some areas of visual science. Important research findings that could benefit the public are routinely ignored or suppressed by the eye care establishment, whose primary concern is to maintain high income levels from prescribing and selling corrective lenses.

By the 1920s, in the midst of these early battles and the growing popularity of the Bates method, optometry was searching for a direction in which to develop. Major discoveries were made about the visual system and the role of the eye muscles and their effect on sight, and an intellectual giant emerged who would revolutionize optometry's concept of vision.

Born in Nebraska at the turn of the nineteenth century, Arthur Martin Skeffington was endowed with an insatiable curiosity and a passion for discipline and logic. After studying for the priesthood, he became an optometrist and probed the mysteries of vision with a religious zeal—showing little regard for money or peer pressure.

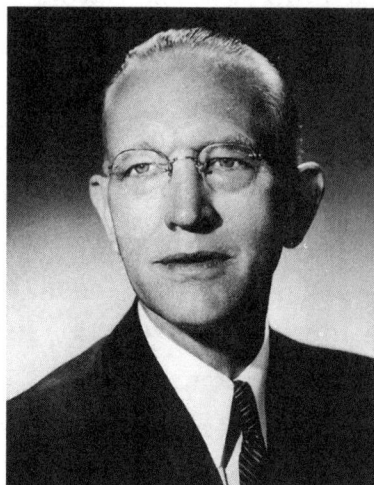

Discoveries of a Doubting Doctor

Dissatisfied with the traditional theory of vision—that the eyes automatically see whatever is in front of them—and the treatment procedures then in use, Skeffington made many important discoveries and laid the foundation of behavioral optometry.

Skeffington was a brilliant, dynamic speaker who traveled widely throughout the United States for almost 40 years, sharing his discoveries and theories with other optometrists. In 1926, he gave a lecture in Kansas City where he met E. B. Alexander, a young optometrist who insisted that the new ideas be made known to his colleagues in Oklahoma.

The 1920s was a period of intense interest in eye exercises and vision improvement due to the Bates method, which undoubtedly influenced Skeffington and Alexander. However, they did not give Bates any recognition or acknowledge his influence, presumably to avoid censorship and ostracism by the eye care establishment.

Nevertheless, Alexander realized that important new discoveries about the visual system were being made, and that optometry needed a program of research and postgraduate education. He joined forces with Skeffington, and in 1928, they established an organization known as the Optometric Extension Program (OEP).

Vision Is a Set of Functions

For the next few decades, Skeffington and Alexander traveled incessantly, recruiting other optometrists and experts in allied disciplines such as psychology and neuroscience who could help behavioral optometry expand its knowledge base and procedures. They discovered that vision comprises more than a dozen different functions, including but not limited to:

- **Acuity:** The ability to see clearly.

- **Accommodation:** The ability to change focus.

- **Fixations:** The ability to maintain a steady gaze on a single object.

- **Saccades:** The ability to make rapid eye movements that abruptly change the point of fixation.

- **Pursuits:** The ability to make smooth, continuous eye movements that enable tracking a moving object.

- **Convergence:** The ability to point the eyes at the same object at the same time.

- **Binocularity:** The ability to use both eyes together to see a single, three-dimensional image.

- **Depth perception:** The ability to judge the distance of objects.

- **Peripheral vision:** The ability to see things without looking directly at them.

From its modest origins in Oklahoma with a membership of 51 optometrists, the OEP spread to every state in the United States and all the Canadian provinces. Today, the OEP has more than 10,000 members worldwide.

Meeting of the Minds

The conceptual foundation of behavioral optometry is that vision is learned during childhood and can be improved with eye exercises and other techniques known as *optometric visual training*. Many behavioral optometrists use some of the Bates exercises such as Palming, Swinging, and Edging, but the OEP has never endorsed the Bates method or given Bates any recognition.

Throughout its history, the OEP has kept an *open door* policy, recognizing that segments of knowledge about the visual system overlap between behavioral optometry and other disciplines such as psychology and ergonomics. As a result, many scientists joined forces with the OEP and made important contributions.

A key figure in the OEP's development was Samuel Renshaw, a psychologist at Ohio State University. Beginning in 1940 and for the next 24 years, he held an annual conference where he invited other psychologists to meet with Skeffington and other behavioral optometrists. These conferences were a melting pot of ideas that generated many important concepts, discoveries, and techniques.

The Crucible of Conception

During that period, behavioral optometry made other important discoveries. Ophthalmologist Arnold Gesell and optometrist Gerald Getman unraveled the mystery of children's vision at the Yale Clinic of Child Development. They discovered the existence of developmental visual problems, revealing how many children have 20/20 acuity but are poor readers. The 1950s also brought major advances through the work of Darell Boyd Harmon, who established the connection between vision and posture.

Internationally acclaimed stress pioneer Hans Selye also played an important role, showing that the visual system could adapt to long periods of reading and close work in a negative and potentially harmful way.

Young, Eskimos, and Chimpanzees

No chronicle of behavioral optometry would be complete without mentioning the pioneering work of Francis Young, a distinguished research scientist at Washington State University and a coauthor of the Power Vision Program.

During the 1960s and 1970s, Young carried out major research into the cause of myopia. At that time, the Eskimos (Inuits) in Barrow, Alaska, were being integrated into mainstream America.

This provided a unique opportunity to test the genetic theory of poor vision. The parents were illiterate, whereas their children were the first generation to go through school. According to the genetic theory, the childrens' and parents' visual systems should be almost identical, with little or no myopia.

Young led a research team to Alaska to study these families. What he discovered stunned the eye care profession. Of 130 parents, 128 had excellent distance vision and 2 had myopia. This was expected because the tribe was living the typical Eskimo lifestyle of hunting and fishing. One parent had −0.25D, and the other, who was the tribe's record keeper, had −1.50D.

On the other hand, 58 percent of the children showed signs of myopia! This was about the same rate of myopia in children in the lower states. Similar investigations were carried out in Micronesia involving native populations and yielded similar findings: Children exposed to the American school system tend to become myopic.

Young concluded that heredity is not a major factor in myopia, and confirmed his findings with studies of chimpanzees, which have eyes that are almost identical to those of humans, and studies of identical twins. Young found that when the chimpanzees looked at close objects, the pressure inside their eyeballs increased, causing them to gradually stretch and deform, producing myopia and other conditions.

Young published 120 research papers on myopia and was honored with the American Optometric Association's prestigious Apollo Award. His findings have been confirmed by numerous other researchers, although many traditional eye care professionals have been taught and still believe that myopia is inherited.

Explosion of Knowledge

As in other branches of science, the winds of change swept through behavioral optometry after the Second World War and brought an abundance of new discoveries and techniques. As the information age dawned, Skeffington realized that the brain functions like a computer and that the principles of information processing could be applied to the visual system.

As behavioral optometrists developed more sophisticated therapy techniques, they were able to prevent and cure a wider range of visual problems. In addition, they were able to help people with normal vision develop superior abilities. Nowadays, behavioral optometrists work closely with professional athletes, training America's sports stars to gain the extra edge vital for success.

Optometric Visual Training

Usually referred to as *visual training*, this is the branch of vision therapy that uses lenses, prisms, or optical devices, often together with eye exercises, to develop or enhance visual abilities. Patients often wear *training lenses* while doing the exercises and *therapeutic lenses* to improve the function of their visual systems.

Behavioral optometrists avoid using the term *eye exercises* in connection with optometric visual training. That's because the term *exercise* implies stronger and more powerful muscles, and the eye muscles, especially the extraocular muscles, don't need strengthening. The goal of optometric visual training is to reprogram the brain to control the eye muscles more efficiently.

> **The goal of vision therapy eye exercises is to improve the function of the visual system, not just to see more clearly.**

The first optometric visual training procedures were developed at the end of the nineteenth century by the French ophthalmologist Emile Javal for treating strabismus (crossed eyes). This was a major breakthrough because most doctors thought that strabismus was inherited and incurable except by means of surgery.

The Roaring Twenties

Stimulated by the success of these early procedures, doctors began to search for new exercises to treat other visual problems. By the 1920s, several different systems were in use. Although the Bates method was the most prolific, other doctors including optometrists T. J. Arneson and R. M. Peckham made important contributions.

Skeffington stimulated the development of many new techniques. In 1937, optometrists George Crow and Harry Fuong published a classic series of papers that integrated optometric visual training with the theoretical concepts of the OEP. Many of the techniques now in use date back to that period.

During the last few decades, a lot of clinical and scientific research has been published on eye exercises and related phenomena. Unfortunately, most of the research has been published in journals that the majority of traditional eye care professionals do not read, such as psychology, ergonomics, and behavioral science journals.

As a result, it usually takes decades for research findings to make their way into the courses that are taught at most optometric colleges and medical schools. Hence the majority of traditional eye care professionals are unaware of the advances that have been made. Analysis of the research yields the following conclusions:

- **The old theory that poor vision is inherited is flawed and must be modified.** Although heredity plays a role in some cases, other factors such as nearpoint stress and the potentially harmful effects of corrective lenses are usually more important. As discussed earlier, the vast majority of visual problems begin with nothing more serious than a minor focusing error.

- **All the visual functions can be improved by means of eye exercises.** Most common visual problems can be prevented. Where visual problems have already occurred, good vision can often be completely or partially restored.

- **Successful visual training usually includes a program of eye exercises to do at home.** This yields faster improvement and helps patients transfer the results to their everyday activities as new visual habits.

Modern Developments

Over the years, the effectiveness of vision therapy has been the subject of intense controversy. The first reason is that major improvements in acuity—the clear flashes—often occur without any changes in refractive error. Although this phenomenon has puzzled many scientists and eye care professionals, the acuity improvement mechanisms are now reasonably well understood (Section 9).

The second reason is the multibillion-dollar eye care industry. If bad eyesight is inherited, nothing can be done except prescribe a lifetime of corrective lenses. On the other hand, if bad eyesight can be improved with vision therapy, eye care professionals are faced with a moral obligation to try to cure their patients, or at least prevent their visual problems from getting worse.

Realistically, however, most people with poor vision are too lazy, ignorant, or apathetic to do eye exercises. All they want is a quick fix, which corrective lenses conveniently provide. If their vision gets worse, they are content to get stronger prescriptions. If they develop cataracts, glaucoma, or retinal detachment, they believe that surgery will provide a quick fix and that the disease will be nothing more than a minor inconvenience.

To give credit where credit is due, the optical glass industry and the eye care establishment have provided hundreds of millions of people with a convenient, affordable quick fix. The traditional method of prescribing corrective lenses has helped and will continue to help many people enjoy happier and more productive lives, even though better methods of vision care are now available.

Vision therapy has come a long way since the Second World War, and eye exercises have been developed that are easier and more effective. Clinical experience has also shown that vision therapy can work for people of all ages. As optometrist Bruce Wick stated:

"Elderly patients are able to learn therapy procedures easily and carry them out more faithfully than children. The usual practice of reserving vision therapy for children can no longer be justified."

Professor Allen, coauthor of the Power Vision Program, also stated:

"No matter how bad your eyesight, vision therapy eye exercises can improve it."

Likewise, in a stunning indirect confirmation of the Bates method, Edward Friedman, professor of optometry at the State University of New York, concluded:

> "Time without glasses is the simplest, most effective, and most important of all visual training exercises. We do not want to return to heavy reliance on glasses. If time without glasses becomes a habit, there will be a real improvement in the clarity of your vision."

Acupressure Exercises from China

One of the most exciting developments in vision therapy came from the People's Republic of China. In the early part of the twentieth century, studies showed that the Chinese were the most myopic people in the world. Following his ascent to power in 1949, Mao Tse-tung ordered acupressure exercises to be used in schools, offices, and factories, In the 1970s, rumors began to circulate among the American eye care profession that this bold experiment had succeeded. In 1976, optometrist Elwin Marg went on a fact-finding mission to China. Upon his return, he reported:

> "Among 1,400 schoolchildren, no spectacles were observed. In the factories, most of the young workers also wore no spectacles."

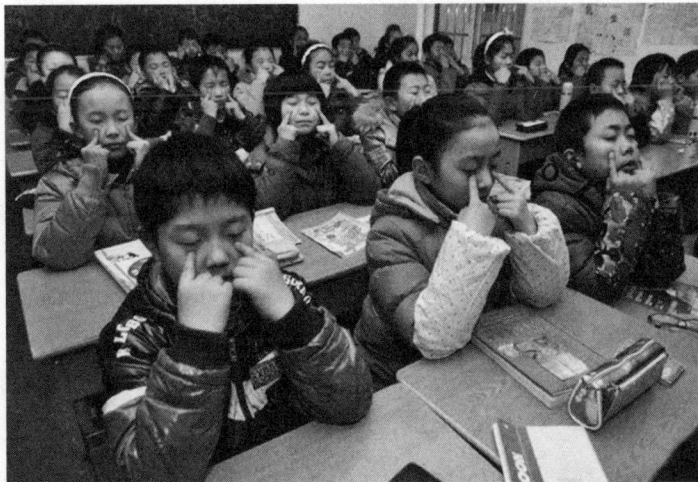

Three years later, behavioral optometrist Paul Harris went to China and brought back the acupressure exercises included in the Power Vision Program. Harris observed:

"In preventive vision care, the Chinese are years ahead of the U.S. By reducing stress, the exercises decrease the pressure inside the eyeball and stop it from deforming."

Peer Pressure and Tradition

By now you're probably asking, "If vision therapy is so effective, why haven't I heard of it before?" There are several reasons why this important treatment procedure has been slow in coming to public attention.

Although many optometrists tried vision therapy after the Second World War, the exercises then available were time-consuming and unprofitable. As a result, most optometrists went back to the old way of prescribing corrective lenses.

Moreover, vision therapy has met with opposition from the optical industry and the eye care establishment. Many ophthalmologists who profit from strabismus surgery were also quick to condemn it. And as previously discussed, a lot of important research has been published in journals that traditional eye doctors do not read.

Consequently, in order to avoid harassment and persecution by the eye care establishment, behavioral optometrists have avoided sensationalism. Although they have helped many patients regain natural, healthy vision—often using the Bates method—they have done so quietly and without seeking attention.

Problems with the Educational System

Almost all optometric colleges were created by or receive funding from the optical glass industry. Consequently, many professors and administrators have been reluctant to accept vision therapy. As behavioral optometrist Burton Worrell recalls:

"In 1968, I became aware of the teachings of Skeffington while completing my degree at UC Berkeley School of Optometry. As president of the student optometric association, I invited him to come and give a lecture.

The arrangements were made and Skeffington was due to appear, but the Dean of the faculty refused to allow him on campus. This incident opened my eyes to the long-standing conflicts within the eye care profession."

Fortunately, the eye care profession is evolving and some positive changes have taken place in the educational system. As a result, most optometric colleges now teach some of the basic exercises, primarily for the treatment of lazy eye and strabismus.

Summary and Conclusion

Although his theory of accommodation was incorrect, Bates must be given credit as the founding father of modern vision therapy. Simply put, he was the originator of the concept that common visual problems can be improved by means of exercise, and an abundance of clinical research has shown this concept to be correct.

The Bates method is most effective against stress-related visual problems. The basic exercises—Palming, Swinging, and Edging—have proved their value for more than a century and are used by many behavioral optometrists as part of their arsenal of therapeutic procedures.

Following in Bates's footsteps, Skeffington and Alexander were the founding fathers of behavioral optometry. They and their colleagues discovered that vision is a set of abilities that are learned during childhood, and that the abilities can be improved by means of eye exercises and other techniques known as optometric visual training.

In contrast to the Bates method, which concentrates on acuity improvement and the reduction of dependence on corrective lenses, optometric visual training improves the performance of the entire visual system.

The OEP (*www.oepf.org*) and OVRA (*www.covd.org*) have a combined membership of more than 12,000 behavioral optometrists and provide referrals to members of the public.

SECTION

7

ADDITIONAL THERAPEUTIC EXERCISES

The following exercises are from the Bates method and optometric visual training.

But first, a few words about behavioral optometry. This is a system of vision care based on the understanding that vision is much more than just seeing clearly. It is a holistic process of vision improvement that helps people understand what they see and interact more effectively with the world.

In contrast to the Bates method, which only improves acuity, behavioral optometry uses vision therapy eye exercises and other procedures known as *optometric visual training* to improve other visual functions and produce a more balanced, accurate, and efficient visual system.

Here are some Bates exercises and optometric visual training exercises. Although they are not part of the dynamic core of the Power Vision Program, you may find some of them helpful, in which case you can add them to your routine or do them as needed.

Swinging

What It Does: This is one of the Bates method exercises. Bates discovered that gently swinging the body from side to side can produce a state of deep relaxation, which he considered to be the basis of natural vision improvement.

Swinging can produce a pleasant state of deep relaxation similar to that produced by hypnosis, often resulting in improved acuity. Swinging may also trigger alpha waves in the brain.

How to Do It: Stand with your feet shoulder-width apart near a chair so you can steady yourself if you lose your balance. Breathe slowly and deeply and let your arms hang loosely; then gently swing back and forth from one side to the other. Keep your eyes open and don't look at anything in particular. Blink every few seconds to keep your eyes lubricated.

Keep the movement going in time to your natural body rhythm. Allow your arms to fly away from your body. You can raise each heel as you swing, but not the entire foot.

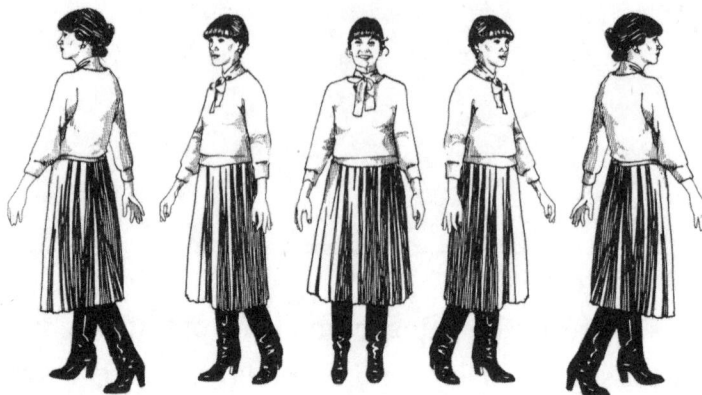

As you swing, the world will appear to swoosh past you. Don't try to look at anything in particular. In the beginning you may become dizzy, in which case close your eyes and stop swinging. When the dizziness subsides, resume the exercise. We recommend doing Swinging for at least 10 minutes. Many people enjoy the sensation and do it for longer as a form of meditation.

Once you've mastered Swinging, try this variation. Put one of the Biofeedback Charts on the wall where you can momentarily see it at the end of each swing. Then try to read the smallest line you can see.

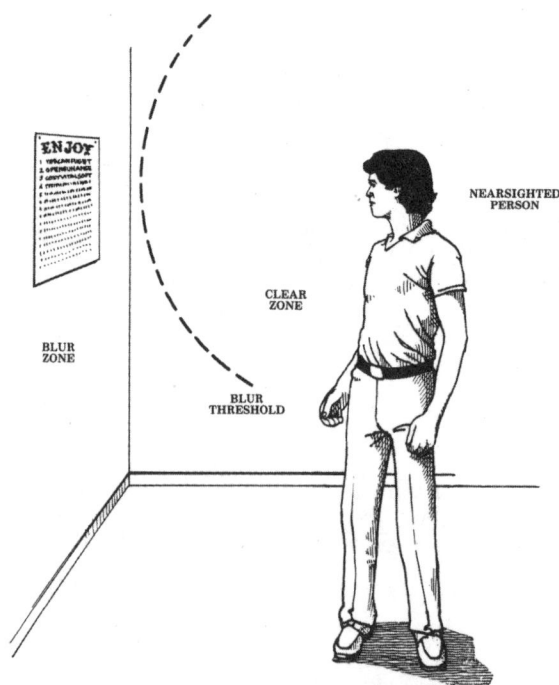

Sunning

What It Does: This is another Bates technique. Bathing your closed eyes in sunlight or a bright indoor light stimulates and relaxes the visual system.

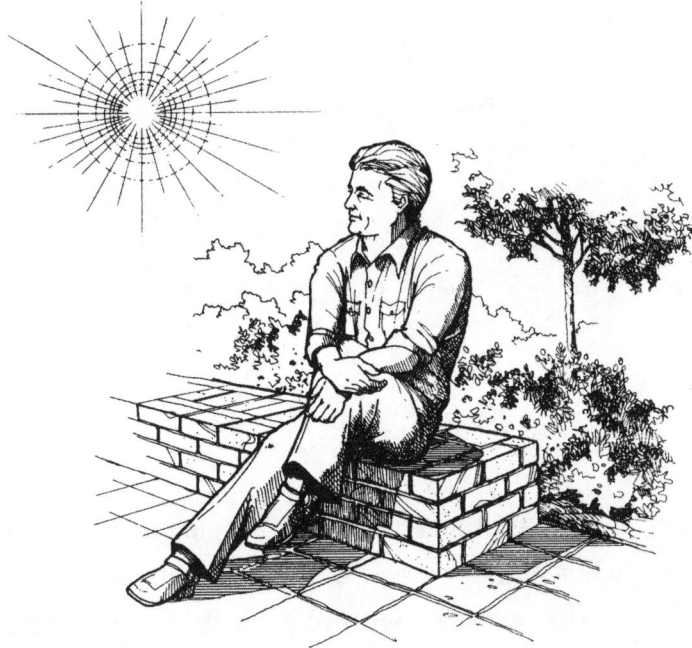

How to Do It: Sit comfortably in bright sunlight or a bright indoor light with your eyes closed.

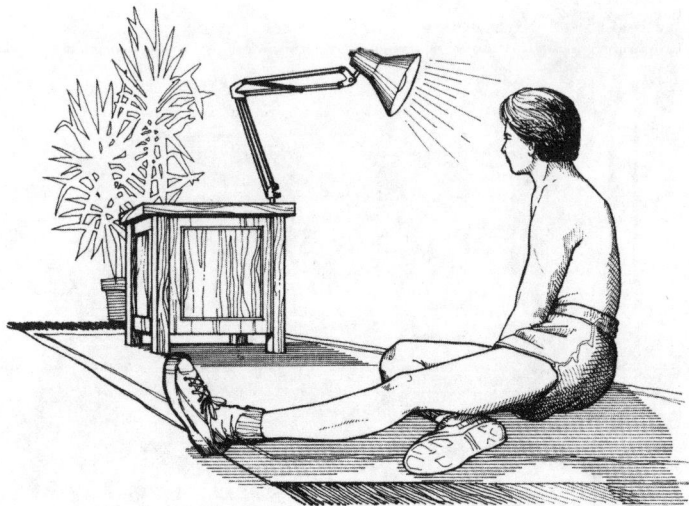

Edging

What It Does: This is another Bates exercise. It involves running your gaze along the edges of different objects. This improves eye coordination and can result in improved acuity.

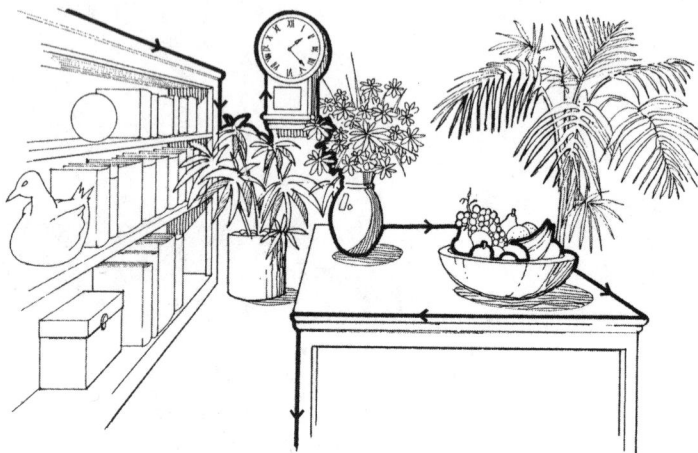

How to Do It: Look at a blurred object and run your gaze along its outline. Follow lines and shapes within the object and progress to smaller and smaller details until you've completely explored it. Do this exercise with objects that are slightly blurred and with objects that are very blurred.

Keep your head still and combine Edging with Squeeze Blinking, Fast Blinking, and Slow Blinking. You may get clear flashes due to a natural contact lens formed from tear fluid.

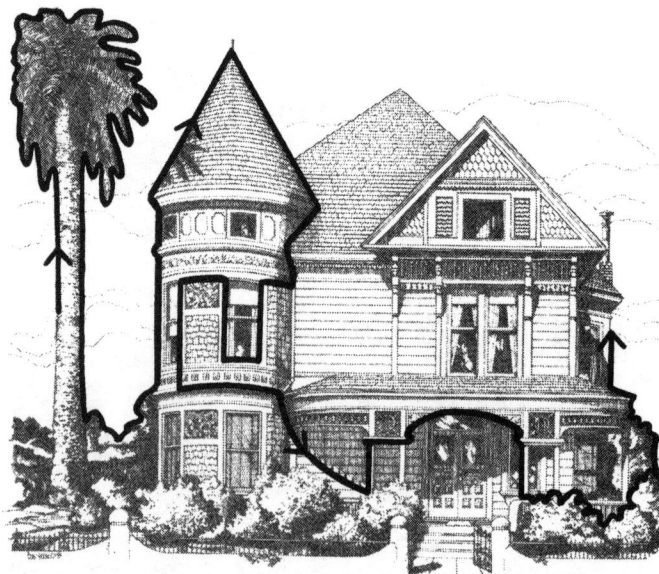

The Windolph Technique

What It Does: This is an eye exercise by Bates practitioner Michael Windolph that improves eye coordination and can trigger clear flashes.

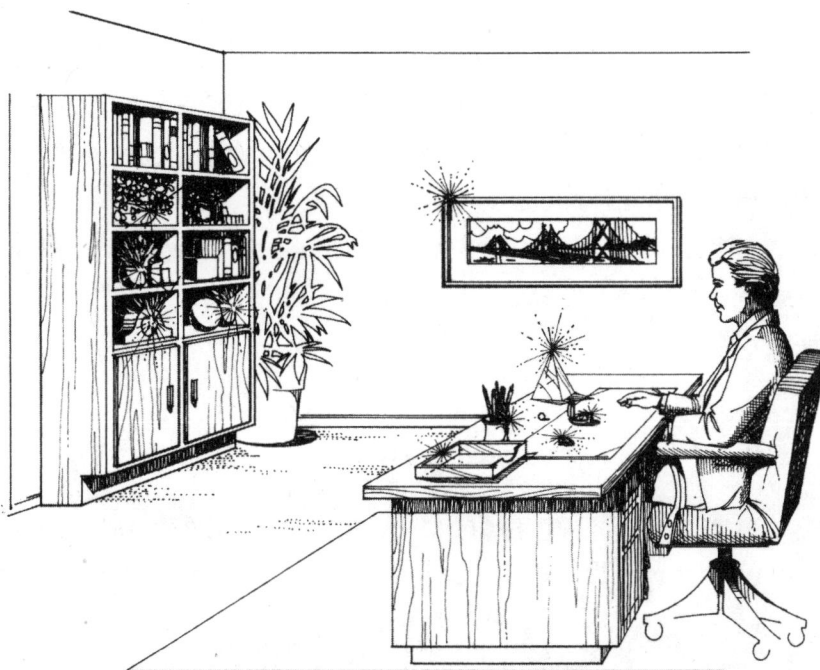

How to Do It: Get some objects with bright reflective surfaces and areas of high contrast such as jewelry, bottles, pieces of aluminum foil, coins, shiny buttons, drinking glasses, Christmas ornaments, toys, and so on. Use interesting objects so you'll enjoy looking at them.

Place these objects at different distances so that they are blurred, and position them so they give lots of reflections and bright spots. Now breathe slowly and deeply. Jump from a bright spot on one object to a bright spot on another object. Run your gaze along the edges of the bright spots and combine this with Squeeze Blinking, Fast Blinking, and Slow Blinking.

If one of the objects or reflections suddenly becomes brighter or clearer, concentrate your entire attention on it. Keep your eyes open and relaxed. Don't squint or strain. The smallest bright spots and reflections are the most likely to trigger clear flashes.

The Bates Method

This was developed by ophthalmologist William Bates around the beginning of the twentieth century and consists of four exercises that are done in this order: **Sunning > Swinging > Palming > Edging**. Bates also recommended looking at small lines on the Snellen eyechart.

Unfortunately, the Bates method can be very time-consuming. Bates recommended doing Swinging and Palming for extended periods of time up to half an hour each. Nevertheless, the Bates method has been used by numerous people for more than 100 years and has proved its effectiveness in many cases.

If you want to try it, we recommend Sunning for 5 minutes, followed by 10 minutes of Swinging, followed by 15 minutes of Palming, followed by 10 minutes of Edging. Instead of Edging different objects, you can use a Biofeedback Chart or the Windolph Technique.

Screening

What It Does: Watching a slightly blurred TV screen can be an effortless and enjoyable way to expand your clear zone. This exercise helps the eyes clear up slightly blurred images.

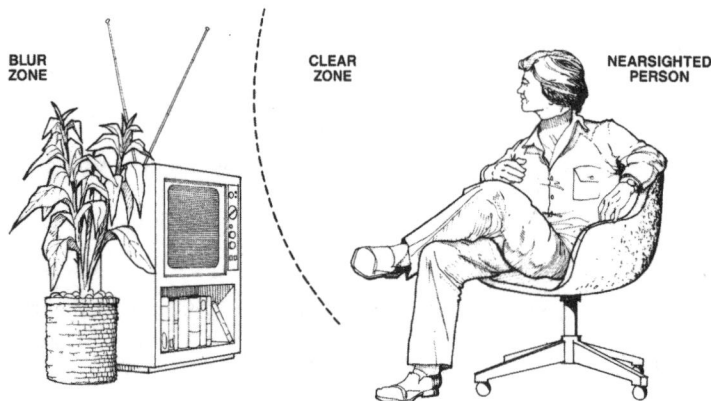

How to Do It: Adjust the TV so that it has areas of high contrast and bright details. Then sit where the screen is slightly blurred. If you are very nearsighted or slightly hyperopic or presbyopic, you may need to sit close to the screen.

Then run your gaze along the edges of areas of high contrast and bright details, going to smaller and smaller areas and details. Do this exercise when watching TV, YouTube, or DVDs.

Remember to do plenty of Squeeze Blinking, Fast Blinking, and Slow Blinking, and look away from the screen at regular intervals. When the picture becomes clearer, move your chair so that it stays slightly blurred. In this way, you can spend hours watching your favorite programs and expand your clear zone at the same time!

Brock String

What It Does: This exercise was developed by optometrist Frederick Brock. It improves eye coordination and the ability to see in three dimensions. If you have a weak eye or a lazy eye, the Brock string can really help you and is well worth the time needed to make it.

Some people discover when they do this exercise that they were only seeing in two dimensions without realizing it. They are amazed when a third dimension suddenly appears out of nowhere and the world becomes more solid, bright, and real than they ever thought possible! Try it and see for yourself.

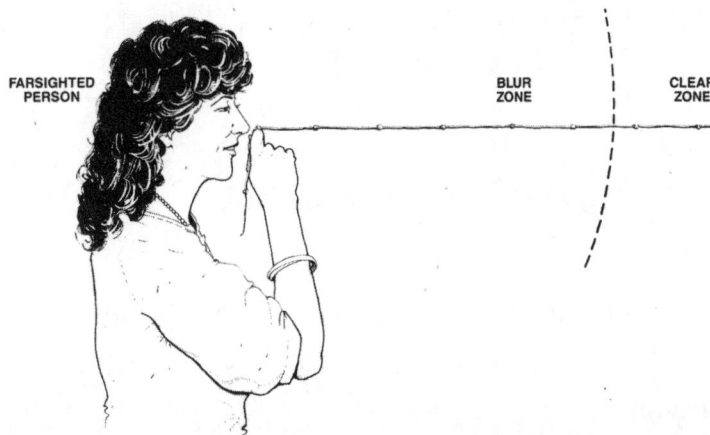

FARSIGHTED PERSON   BLUR ZONE   CLEAR ZONE

How to Do It: Get some thick string about 12 feet long, and tie beads or large knots every 6 inches. Fasten one end of the string to a doorknob or hook on the wall. Hold the other end to your nose.

Focus on one bead at a time. You should see two strings—one from each eye—crossing and forming an "X" at the bead. If one string is much fainter than the other, it means that you have an abnormally weak eye or a lazy eye.

Start by looking at the bead closest to you; then gradually move to the beads farther away, one bead at a time. Don't rush. Allow the "X" to settle until it is completely stable. If one of the strings is much fainter than the other one, focus your attention on it and mentally try to bring it up to the level of the other string without straining, squinting, or tricks. Then move to the next bead. Go back and forth along the string, and blink every few seconds to keep your eyes lubricated.

Marsden Ball

What It Does: This exercise was developed by optometrist William Marsden. It improves eye tracking, hand-eye coordination, and accommodation.

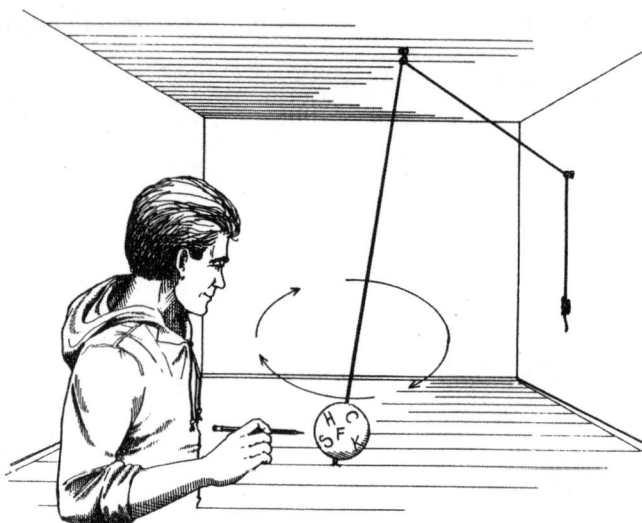

How to Do It: Hang some string from the ceiling and fasten a ball to the end. Write letters on the ball. Now swing the ball to and fro. Try to touch the middle of any letter when the ball is near you.

You can also do the exercise lying on your back with the ball directly above you, in which case follow the ball with your eyes without trying to touch it.

Finger Jumps

What It Does: This exercise improves saccadic eye movements, improves extraocular muscle coordination, and checks for glaucoma.

How to Do It: Put on some music. Then make two relaxed fists with pointed fingers, and let your eyes jump from one finger to the other in time to the beat. Keep your head still. Vary the distance and position of your fingers.

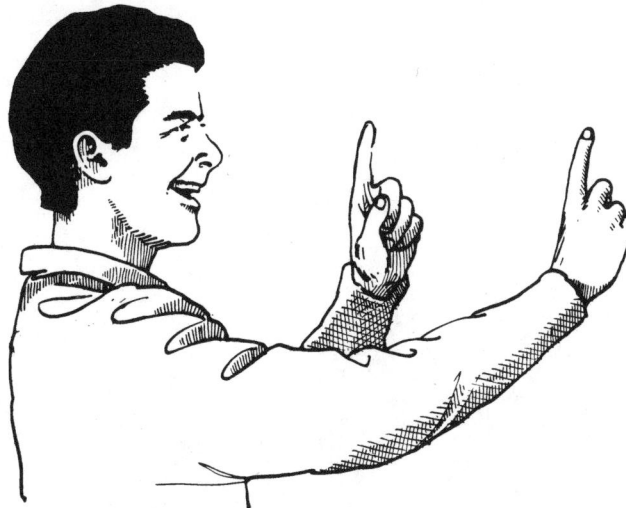

Blink every few seconds to keep your eyes lubricated:

up > down > sideways > front > back > farther apart > closer together >
front > back > up > down > sideways > front > back > farther apart >
closer together > front > back > . . .

An important variation is to improve your peripheral vision. Put a large dot on the wall and look at it. Hold your fingers at arm's length in line with the dot. Then slowly move your arms apart. Keep looking at the dot and wiggle your fingers. See how far apart you can go. Repeat the exercise and move your arms upwards, downwards, then diagonally.

If your vision does not go all the way to the extreme edge of your arm movements, it may be a sign of glaucoma or retinal detachment, in which case you should immediately have your eyes examined by an eye care professional, preferably an ophthalmologist. Don't wait or make excuses. Don't think it's not a big thing. If you have either of these diseases, they must be treated without delay or you risk further loss of vision.

Tossing

What It Does: This simple exercise improves accommodation, pursuits, and hand-eye coordination.

How to Do It: Toss the ball from one hand to the other. Keep your eyes on the ball at all times. Blink every few seconds to keep your eyes lubricated.

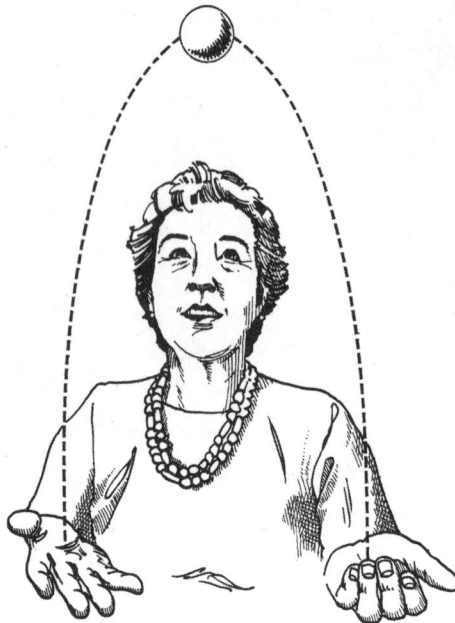

Balancing

What It Does: This exercise requires an eye patch and coordinates your visual field with your position in it. It is especially important for older people.

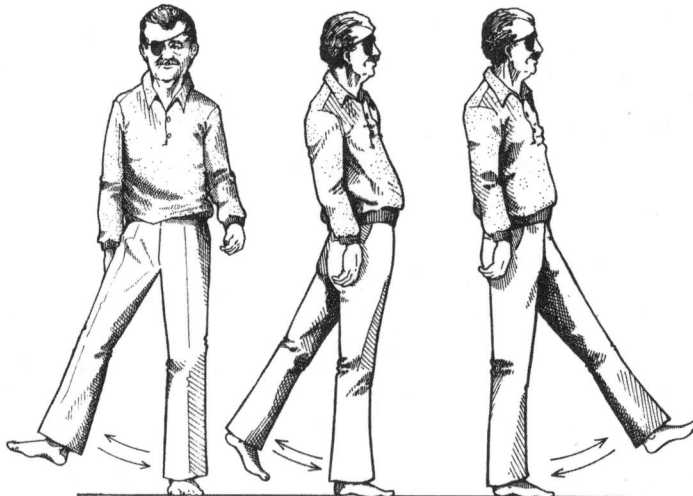

How to Do It: Stand on one leg with one of your eyes patched and look at an object across the room. Now slowly move the other leg in different directions. Repeat the exercise with the other leg and with the other eye patched. Keep a chair nearby to help you steady yourself if you lose your balance. Blink every few seconds to keep your eyes lubricated.

Blocking

What It Does: This exercise improves peripheral vision.

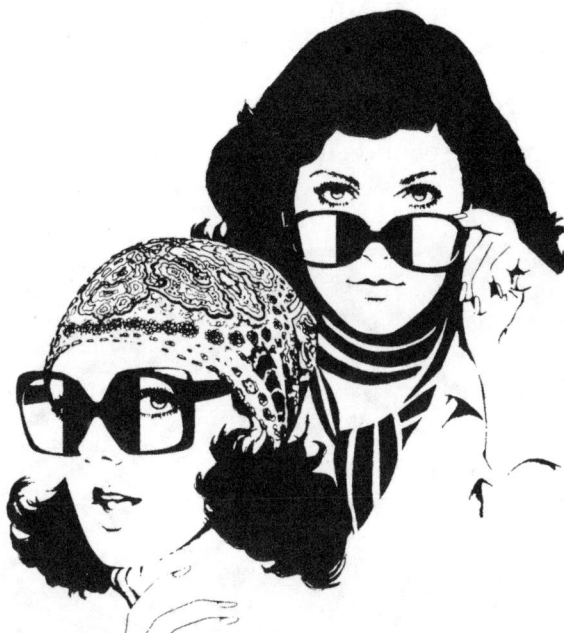

How to Do It: Use spectacles or sunglasses. Cover part of the lenses next to your nose with adhesive tape so your central vision is obscured. You can do this exercise for long periods of time during normal activities. Don't do it in potentially dangerous situations such as driving, crossing the street, or using kitchen utensils or power tools.

Dish Rotations

What It Does: It improves pursuits and eye-hand coordination.

How to Do It: Put a marble or a small piece of fruit such as a grape or cherry in a baking dish; then slowly roll it around. Keep your eyes on the marble or piece of fruit at all times. Blink every few seconds to keep your eyes lubricated.

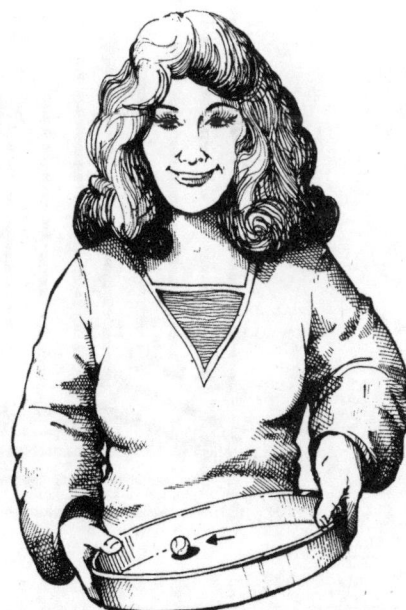

Scanning Chart

What It Does: It improves saccades and fixation.

How to Do It: Follow the line from A to B one dot at a time. Don't rush. Look directly at each dot for about a second; then move to the next dot. You can put the chart where it is clear or slightly blurred. You may get an improvement in acuity if you do it when it is slightly blurred. Blink every few seconds to keep your eyes lubricated.

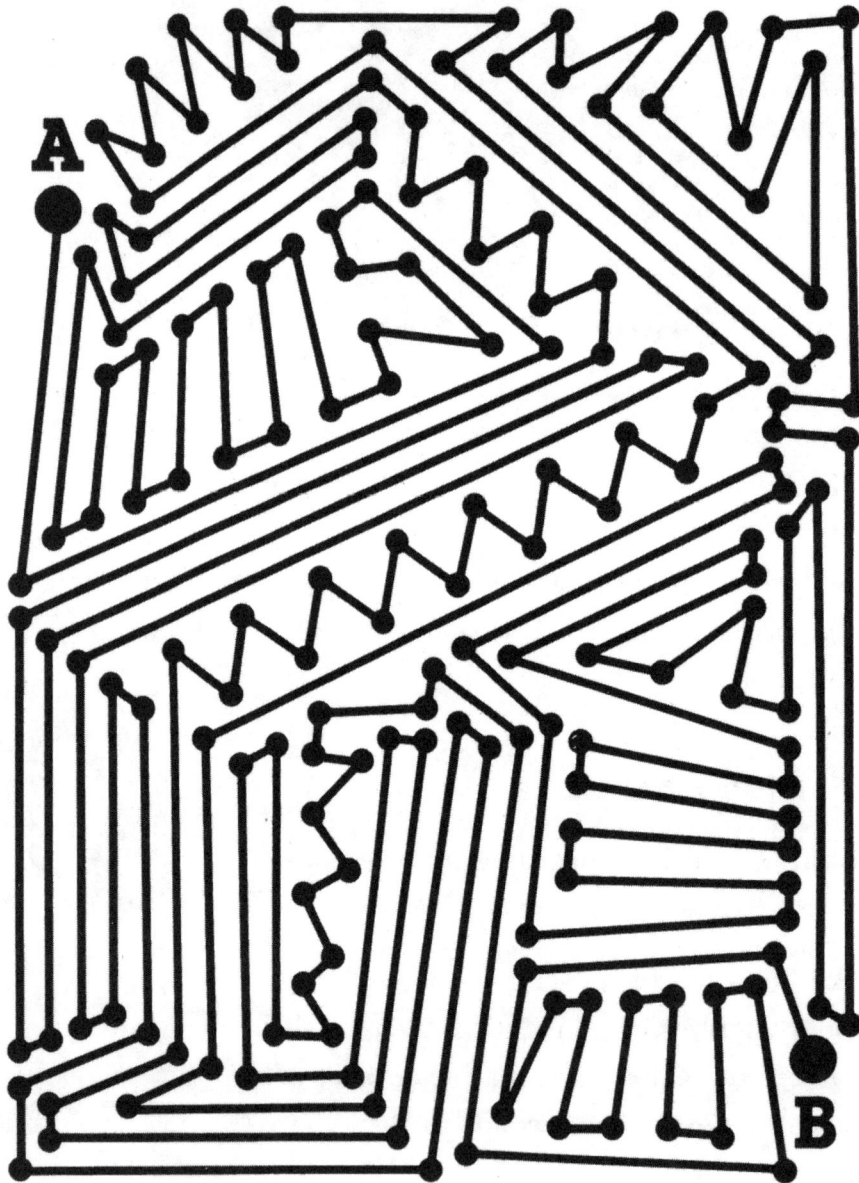

Labyrinth

What It Does: This exercise improves pursuits and eye tracking.

How to Do It: Follow the line from the outer dot to the center. Keep your eyes on the line at all times. You can put the chart where it is completely clear or slightly blurred. You may get an improvement in acuity if you do it when it is slightly blurred. Blink every few seconds to keep your eyes lubricated.

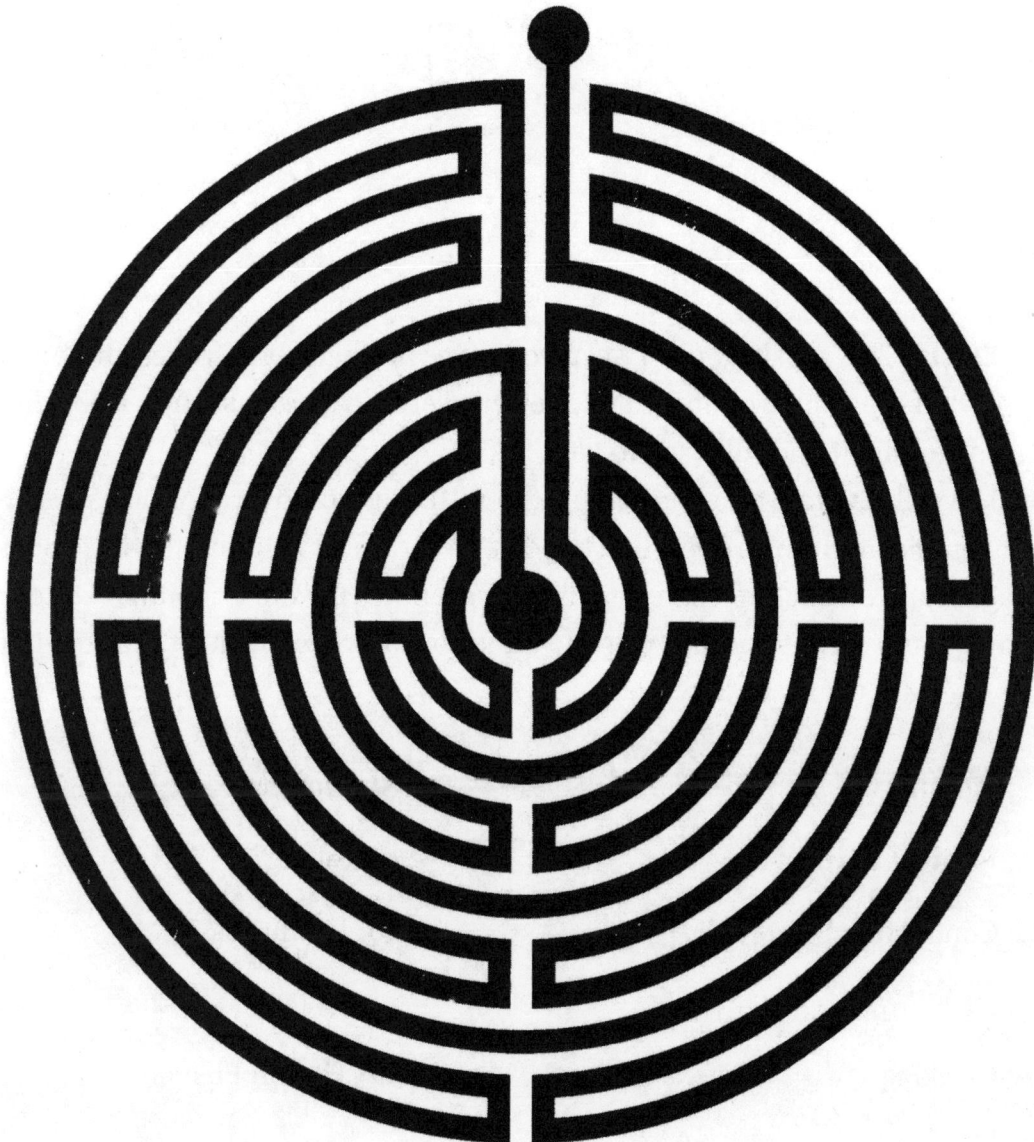

THE PERSEVERANCE CASINO

What It Does: It improves accommodation, pursuits, and motivation.

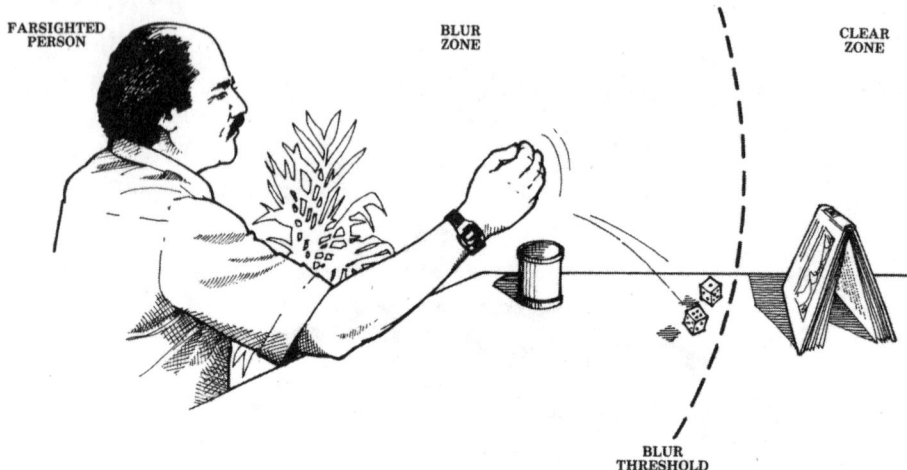

How to Do It: Toss a pair of dice. Keep your eyes on them at all times and blink every few seconds to keep your eyes lubricated. You can set up a barrier such as a book or a box, which the dice will hit and roll back to you.

The dice will generate numbers from 2 (1 +1) through 12 (6 + 6). Assign an exercise to each number and do the exercise when the dice stop rolling. After doing the exercise, roll the dice again and do another exercise. The Perseverance Casino is an interesting and fun way of doing the exercises because you don't know what will come next. Use the following sequence or create your own list:

- 2: Palming
- 3: Fusion Chart
- 4: Conducting
- 5: Detailing
- 6: Clocking
- 7: Flexing

- 8: Blinking
- 9: Rolling
- 10: Pushups
- 11: Biofeedback Chart
- 12: Thumb Fusion

SECTION

8

COMMON VISUAL PROBLEMS

This section briefly summarizes and explains common visual problems, including amblyopia (lazy eye), asthenopia (eyestrain), astigmatism, cataracts, color blindness (color vision deficiency), computer vision syndrome, diabetic retinopathy, dry eye disease, floaters, glaucoma, hyperopia (farsightedness), macular degeneration, myopia (nearsightedness), pink eye (conjunctivitus), presbyopia (aging eyes), retinal detachment, and strabismus (crossed eyes).

For more information, go to the following websites:

- **American Optometric Association (www/aoa.org).** Provides guidelines and resources for the diagnosis and traditional methods of treating common visual problems.

- **Optometric Extension Program Foundation (www.oepf.org).** Provides referrals to members of the public and educational resources to eye care professionals.

- **Optometric Vision Development & Rehabilitation Association (www.covd.org).** Provides referrals to members of the public and educational resources to eye care professionals.

Some Hard Facts About Eye Disease

There are approximately 77 million Americans over 60 years old. According to the National Eye Institute, approximately 24 million have cataracts, 3 million have glaucoma, 21 million have macular degeneration, and 10 million have diabetic retinopathy. Although these statistics include diseases in their early stages, it means that if you rely on traditional eye care, there's a 75% chance that you'll develop one of them as you grow older.

Of course, the aging process is often a factor whether or not you wear corrective lenses. However, common sense dictates that you should do everything possible to minimize the risk. Although most eye care professionals don't discuss these statistics with patients, we believe that you need to know the facts so that you can make an informed decision about how your eyes should be treated.

Don't make the mistake of assuming that you'll always be able to see. Really effective eye care is much more than just selecting fashionable frames to go with stronger lenses or assuming that if you develop an eye disease, drugs or surgery will somehow fix it.

Although traditional eye care has helped millions of people lead happier, more productive lives, and will continue to do so in the future, much more can be done. Vision therapy eye exercises increase the flow of blood and nutrients to the eyes, making them healthier and reducing the risk of disease.

The Power Vision Program contains the best of these exercises, so don't just read it and put it away. Use it and know that you are doing everything possible to make your eyes healthier and enjoy a lifetime of better vision.

Now for information about common visual problems.

Amblyopia (Lazy Eye)

Amblyopia, also known as *lazy eye*, is a vision development disorder where an eye fails to achieve normal visual acuity, even with glasses or contact lenses. It usually affects only one eye and is a common cause of poor vision in children that can have a significant impact on daily life if left untreated.

Causes
Amblyopia typically develops before the age of six. Several factors can contribute to its development, including:

- **Strabismus.** Misalignment of the eyes, where one eye turns in, out, up, or down.

- **Refractive errors.** A significant difference in the refractive errors (nearsightedness, farsightedness, or astigmatism) between the two eyes.

- **Visual deprivation.** A common cause is placing a child's crib next to a wall. One eye sees the wall, whereas the other eye is visually stimulated by the world around it.

- **Family history.** A genetic predisposition to eye conditions.

- **Premature birth.** Babies born prematurely are at higher risk.

Symptoms

Amblyopia may not always be obvious. Some signs include favoring one eye over the other, squinting or tilting the head to one side, and bumping into objects on one side.

Diagnosis/Treatment

Early diagnosis is crucial for effective treatment, although adults with amblyopia can also benefit from treatment. Children should have a comprehensive eye exam when they are six months old and again at three years old. Treatment options for amblyopia include:

- **Prescription lenses.** Glasses or contact lenses to correct refractive errors.

- **Eye patching.** Covering the stronger eye to force the weaker eye to work harder.

- **Vision therapy.** Exercises and activities designed to improve coordination and focus between the eyes.

- **Prisms.** Special lenses that help align the images seen by each eye.

Prevention

Regular eye exams and early intervention are essential. Parents should make sure their children receive comprehensive eye exams at the recommended ages and seek treatment if any issues are detected.

Management

If left untreated, amblyopia can lead to permanent vision loss in the lazy eye. It can also affect self-esteem and social interactions due to the cosmetic appearance of strabismus or the functional limitations of reduced vision. However, with proper treatment, many children—and adults—can achieve significant improvements in vision.

Vision Therapy for Amblyopia

Amblyopia is a developmental visual problem that arises during the first few months of life. It is usually caused by one eye not receiving enough visual stimulation to develop properly—such as putting the baby in a crib next to a wall or covering one eye with a blanket for long periods of time.

In such an environment, one eye sees a bright new world of moving shapes and colors, whereas the other eye only sees the wall or the blanket. The result is a highly dominant eye through which the brain does most of its seeing and a lazy eye that the brain ignores. In most cases, there's nothing basically wrong with the lazy eye.

The amblyopic visual system is like a four-cylinder car with two cylinders misfiring. It will consume a lot of fuel and won't go very fast. Likewise, people with amblyopia often have other visual problems, such as defective eye movements, poor eye coordination, and reading disabilities.

It's often possible to bring a lazy eye up to par simply by patching the dominant eye for long periods of time. This forces the brain to use the lazy eye and increase its functionality. For fastest results, we recommend covering the dominant eye with adhesive surgical tape or an adhesive bandage. Do this for several days at a time, such as over the weekend. Do all the Power Exercises with the dominant eye patched or covered.

At first, it will seem weird or uncomfortable having your dominant eye covered, but persevere and you will enter a brighter, more solid visual space. Realize that you are probably not yet seeing in three dimensions because your brain is not using the image from your lazy eye, so bringing your lazy eye up to par can open up a new dimension that you were previously unaware of.

Asthenopia (Eyestrain)

Asthenopia, commonly known as *eyestrain*, is characterized by discomfort and fatigue in the eyes due to prolonged visual tasks at close distances. Asthenopia is becoming increasingly common in our digital age, where many people spend hour after hour looking at computers, tablets, or smartphones.

Causes

Asthenopia can be caused by several different factors, including digital devices or reading or driving for long periods of time. In addition, digital screens often have glare, flicker, and contrast that can contribute to eyestrain. The rate of blinking is also reduced when using digital screens, which can cause dry, irritated eyes.

Under normal conditions, the average person blinks about 15 to 20 times per minute. However, when reading or staring at a computer screen, this rate can drop to about 4 to 8 times per minute.

Symptoms

The symptoms of asthenopia often include:

- **Eye discomfort.** A feeling of dryness, burning, or itching in the eyes.

- **Headaches.** Frequent headaches, especially after prolonged visual tasks.

- **Blurred vision.** Difficulty focusing, especially after extended periods of screen time.

- **Neck and shoulder pain.** Muscle strain from poor posture while using digital devices.

- **Sensitivity to light.** Increased sensitivity to bright lights or glare.

- **Ticks in the eyelids.** Involuntary eyelid movements.

Management

Managing asthenopia involves adopting various strategies to reduce eyestrain and improve visual comfort, including proper ergonomics and regular breaks. Here are some effective management strategies:

- **Ergonomics.** Ensure that your workspace is ergonomically designed. Position your computer screen at eye level and about an arm's length away. Use a chair with good back support to maintain proper posture.

- **20-20-20 rule.** Every 20 minutes, take a 20-second break and look at something 20 feet away. This helps reduce eye fatigue by giving your eyes a chance to relax.

- **Blinking.** Consciously blink more often to keep your eyes moist and prevent dryness.

- **Proper lighting.** Ensure that your workspace is well lit to reduce glare and reflections on your screen.

- **Vision therapy.** Perform eye exercises to relax your eyes and help them focus better.

- **Special glasses.** Consider using glasses with blue light filters or anti-reflective coatings to reduce eyestrain from digital screens.

Conclusion

Asthenopia is a common visual problem that can cause significant discomfort and impact daily life. However, by understanding its causes, recognizing the symptoms, and implementing effective management strategies, individuals can alleviate eyestrain and improve their visual health.

Vision Therapy for Asthenopia

Instead of reading page after page without stopping, or spending hours gazing at a computer screen, take frequent breaks. Close your eyes for a few seconds; then open them and look at a far object or something across the room. Do plenty of blinking to keep your eyes lubricated.

Discipline yourself to take 50 breaks per day and keep a written record using *bars and gates*. Every time you take a break, add a bar to the gate. This simple strategy can cure computer eyestrain and headaches, often within a few days.

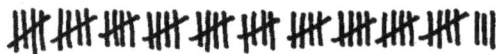

Tape the Reminder Card to your computer. You can also use it as a bookmark. Put it a few pages ahead, and when you reach it, take a break and add a bar to the gate. Then put it a few more pages ahead and continue reading.

When the eyestrain has subsided and your eyes feel comfortable, do all the Power Exercises with emphasis on Flexing, Blinking, Rolling, Detailing, and the Biofeedback Charts. The goal is to increase the flexibility and focusing range of the eye's inner lens and stimulate the production of tear fluid.

Astigmatism

Astigmatism is a common visual problem that causes blurred, distorted, or double vision. It occurs when the cornea or the eye's inner lens has an irregular shape. This prevents light from focusing properly on the retina. Astigmatism is a refractive error that usually affects both eyes. It can occur on its own or combined with other refractive errors such as hyperopia, myopia, or presbyopia. It is not a disease.

Causes

The exact cause of astigmatism is not known, but it is often hereditary or present from birth, when it can be caused by a difficult delivery causing the skull to become distorted. It can also develop after an eye injury, after eye surgery, or due to a disease called *keratoconus*, where the cornea becomes progressively thinner and cone-shaped. Risk factors include a family history of astigmatism, eye injuries, and various eye diseases.

Symptoms

Common symptoms include blurred or distorted vision at any distance; seeing multiple images; headaches, squinting, or difficulty seeing well at night.

Diagnosis

A comprehensive examination by an eye care professional can diagnose astigmatism. The examination usually includes tests such as measuring how well you see letters on a distance chart, measuring the curvature of the cornea, and determining the power of lenses needed to compensate for the refractive error.

Treatment

Astigmatism can be treated with glasses, contact lenses, surgery, or vision therapy. Glasses and contact lenses are the most common methods of treatment and improve the symptoms by focusing light properly on the retina. Refractive surgery, such as LASIK, can reshape the cornea to correct the irregularities causing the astigmatism. In many cases, vision therapy can reduce the amount of astigmatism naturally.

Management

Although there is no way to prevent astigmatism, wearing protective eyewear during sports can reduce the risk. Avoiding eyestrain by taking breaks during prolonged screen time can be beneficial.

Conclusion

Astigmatism is a common vision problem that can cause blurred or distorted vision. It is often hereditary and can be present from birth or develop later in life. It can occur alone or in combination with other refractive errors. With proper diagnosis and treatment, astigmatism can be managed effectively, allowing individuals to enjoy clear and comfortable vision.

Vision Therapy for Astigmatism

Although astigmatism can be inherited, in many cases it seems to be the result of nothing more serious than a bad posture with the head habitually tilted to the side. The reason is that the visual system helps maintain our sense of balance by looking for horizontal features to provide us with a frame of reference. If the head is tilted, the extraocular muscles pull unequally, which causes the eyeball and cornea to go out of shape.

Astigmatism is the most common visual problem because few people have perfect posture. However, it is usually minor and doesn't affect acuity. On the other hand, heavy readers who habitually tilt their head tend to have significant amounts of astigmatism, often combined with myopia.

To improve astigmatism, first determine if your head is tilted. Look in a mirror or ask a friend. If so, cultivate the habit of tilting your head the other way. Write notes to yourself to tilt your head the other way and put them in strategic positions at home, at work, and in your car. If the astigmatism is caused by a head tilt, it will diminish over a period of months. Tilting your head the opposite way will feel weird at first, but you'll soon get used to it.

Even if your head is not habitually tilted, do all the exercises in all the modules. Do extra Clocking and Rolling to help the extraocular muscles optimize their configuration.

Cataracts

Cataracts are a common eye disease that can affect your vision and can result in blindness if untreated. They occur when your eye's inner lens becomes cloudy or opaque. The cloudiness can make things look hazy, blurry, or less colorful.

Causes

The most common cause of cataracts is aging. As we get older, the proteins in the inner lens can break down and cause cloudiness. However, other factors can contribute to the development of cataracts, including:

- **Diabetes.** People with diabetes are at a higher risk for developing cataracts.

- **Medications.** Certain medications, such as corticosteroids, can increase the risk of cataracts.

- **Ultraviolet radiation.** Prolonged exposure to UV rays without protection can increase the likelihood of cataracts.

- **Smoking and alcohol.** Both smoking and excessive alcohol consumption have been linked to an increased risk of cataracts.

- **Nutritional deficiencies.** Low levels of antioxidants, such as vitamins C and E, may be associated with cataract formation.

- **Family history.** If your close relatives have had cataracts, you are more likely to develop them.

Cataracts can develop in different parts of the inner lens, and they are named based on their location:

- **Nuclear cataracts.** These form in the center of the inner lens and can cause the lens to darken and turn yellow or brown.

- **Cortical cataracts.** These affect the outer layer of the inner lens and often look like spokes or wedges.

- **Posterior cataracts.** These form at the back of the inner lens and can cause significant vision problems, especially in bright light.

Symptoms

Common symptoms include blurred or hazy vision, double vision or seeing ghost images, difficulty seeing well at night, colors appearing faded or yellowed, increased sensitivity to bright light and glare.

Diagnosis/Treatment

If you think you have cataracts, it's important to see an eye care professional for a comprehensive eye exam. An eye care professional can diagnose cataracts and recommend appropriate treatment options. In the early stages, stronger glasses or better lighting may help improve vision.

However, if cataracts significantly impair your vision, surgery may be necessary. This involves removing the inner lens and replacing it with an artificial lens. It's a common and usually safe procedure that can restore clear vision.

Management

Although age-related cataracts cannot be prevented, there are steps you can take to reduce your risk:

- **Wear sunglasses.** Protect your eyes from UV rays by wearing sunglasses that block 100% of UV rays.

- **Quit smoking.** Reducing or quitting smoking can lower your risk of developing cataracts.

- **Manage health conditions.** Keep diabetes and other diseases that can lead to cataracts under control.

- **Eat a healthy diet.** A diet rich in antioxidants, such as fruits and vegetables, may reduce the risk of cataracts.

Vision Therapy for Cataracts

Surprisingly, eye exercises can have a major positive impact on cataracts and may partially or completely dissolve them.

The first case that came to our attention was an elderly lady who used eye exercises to reduce her dependency on bifocals. She was scheduled for cataract surgery, and to our amazement, she said that her cataracts had dissolved after doing the eye exercises for two months and she no longer needed the surgery. Her ophthalmologist confirmed her report.

Another patient reported dissolving his cataracts with a flashing light! These and other cases caused us to look closely at the aging mechanism and its impact on the eyes and visual system. Here are our conclusions.

How Aging Affects the Eyes

The eye's inner lens does not contain blood vessels because they would block light and obscure vision. As a result, all the nutrients entering the inner lens come from the surrounding fluids through diffusion. The same process takes place with cellular waste products, which are expelled through diffusion.

Nutrients are pumped into the eye from the posterior base of the ciliary muscle. Cellular waste products are pumped out of the eye through Schlemm's canal, which is located at the anterior base of the iris sphincter muscle. The fluids inside the eye circulate as a result of the ciliary muscle and the iris sphincter muscle expanding and contracting and the inner lens changing its shape.

Like all other bodily tissues, the eye's tissues decline with age. The ciliary muscle and the iris sphincter muscle become less active, and the inner lens loses its flexibility. The flow of nutrients decreases, and cellular waste products are not properly expelled. As a result, the inner lens becomes rigid and unhealthy, which increases the risk of cells dying and forming a cataract.

Vision therapy for cataracts maximizes the action of the ciliary muscle and the iris sphincter muscle. The strategy is to stimulate activity in and around the iris and focusing system.

The goal is to revitalize the cells with a better nutrient flow and flush out toxic waste products and cellular debris, making the inner lens more transparent. Our clinical experience indicates that cataracts can often be improved with vision therapy eye exercises, avoiding or delaying surgery.

We recommend doing all the exercises in the Power Vision Program under the supervision of an eye care professional. Do extra Blinking, Flexing, Pushups, Conducting, Palming, Hydrotherapy, and Light Therapy. Repeat the affirmation "My eyes are getting better and my vision is improving!"

Eat plenty of fruits and vegetables and take a high-quality supplement for the eyes. We recommend Bausch & Lomb's PreserVision (AREDS 2), which contains the formula advocated by the National Eye Institute for reducing the risk of age-related diseases.

Color Blindness (Color Vision Deficiency)

Color blindness, also known as *color vision deficiency*, is a condition where a person is unable to see colors in the usual way. This condition affects how individuals perceive colors, making it difficult to distinguish between certain shades, especially reds and greens. Understanding the causes of color blindness, knowing the symptoms, and using appropriate management strategies can help individuals navigate this condition more effectively.

Causes
Color blindness is usually inherited and is caused by genetic mutations that affect the cones in the retina. Cones are specialized cells responsible for detecting color, and there are three types: red, green, and blue cones.

When one or more of the cones is missing or is not functioning correctly, it results in color vision deficiency. Most cases of color blindness are congenital, meaning individuals are born with it. However, it can also develop later in life due to certain medical conditions or medications.

Symptoms

The symptoms of color blindness can vary in severity. Some individuals have mild symptoms and do not even realize they have the condition, while others may experience more pronounced difficulties. Common symptoms include:

- **Difficulty distinguishing among colors.** Especially red and green, or blue and yellow.

- **Reduced color brightness.** Colors may appear less vibrant or dull.

- **Inability to see certain colors.** In rare cases, individuals may see everything in shades of gray (*achromatopsia*).

- **Quick side-to-side eye movements.** In severe cases, individuals may experience involuntary eye movements known as *nystagmus*.

Management

Although there is no cure for color blindness, there are several strategies to help manage the condition and improve quality of life. These include:

- **Special glasses and contact lenses.** These can help individuals distinguish between colors more effectively.

- **Visual aids.** Using color-coded labels, apps, and other tools can assist in daily activities.

- **Education and awareness.** Learning about the condition and informing others can help create a supportive environment.

Conclusion

Color blindness is a common condition that affects approximately 8% of men and 1% of women. By understanding its causes, recognizing the symptoms, and implementing effective management strategies, individuals can navigate this condition more effectively.

Vision Therapy for Color Blindness

While there are strategies that will help manage color blindness, there are no eye exercises that are effective against it.

Computer Vision Syndrome

Computer vision syndrome (CVS) is a group of vision-related problems resulting from the prolonged use of computers, tablets, e-readers, and smartphones. With the increasing use of digital devices at work and for leisure activities, CVS has become a common issue affecting millions of people worldwide.

Causes

The primary cause of CVS is the extended use of digital screens, which require the eyes to constantly scan the screen and focus on items of interest. This repetitive motion can strain the eye muscles, leading to discomfort and fatigue.

In addition, digital screens often have glare, flicker, and contrast that can contribute to eyestrain. Another factor is that the rate of blinking is significantly reduced when using digital screens, which can cause dry, irritated eyes.

Under normal conditions, the average person blinks about 15 to 20 times per minute. When reading or staring at a computer screen, the rate can drop to about 4 to 8 times per minute.

Symptoms

Common symptoms include:

- **Blurred vision.** Difficulty focusing, especially when shifting focus from near to far objects.

- **Dry, irritated eyes.** Eyes may feel dry, itchy, or burning due to reduced blinking.

- **Headaches.** Frequent headaches, particularly behind the eyes.

- **Neck and shoulder pain.** Poor posture while using digital devices can lead to aches and pains in these areas.

- **Double vision.** Seeing double images, especially when looking at screens for extended periods.

- **Sensitivity to light.** Increased sensitivity to bright lights and glare.

Treatment

For those already experiencing CVS, treatment options include:

- **Vision correction.** Glasses or contact lenses specifically designed for computer use can help reduce eyestrain.

- **Medications.** In some cases, eye drops or medications may be prescribed to manage symptoms.

- **Lifestyle changes**. Incorporating regular breaks, adjusting screen settings, and improving workspace ergonomics can significantly alleviate symptoms.

Prevention/Management

To prevent and manage CVS, use the following strategies:

- **Follow the 20-20-20 rule.** Every 20 minutes, take a 20-second break and look at something 20 feet away. This helps reduce eyestrain.

- **Adjust your screen settings.** Reduce brightness, increase text size, and use a matte screen filter to decrease glare.

- **Maintain proper posture.** Ensure your screen is at eye level and about an arm's length away. Use an ergonomic chair to support your back and neck.

- **Blink more often.** Consciously blink to keep your eyes moist and reduce dryness.

- **Use artificial tears.** Over-the-counter lubricating eye drops can help alleviate dryness.

- **Get regular eye exams.** Visit your eye care professional regularly to ensure your prescription is up-to-date and to check for any underlying eye conditions.

Conclusion

Computer vision syndrome is a common but manageable condition that can affect anyone who spends significant time using digital devices. By taking proactive steps to adjust your screen habits and environment, you can reduce the risk of CVS and maintain healthy eyes.

Vision Therapy for CVS

Instead of reading page after page without stopping, or spending hours gazing at a computer screen, take frequent breaks. Close your eyes for a few seconds, and then open them and look at a far object or something across the room. Do plenty of blinking to keep your eyes lubricated.

Discipline yourself to take 50 breaks per day and keep a written record using *bars and gates*. Every time you take a break, add a bar to the gate. This simple strategy can cure CVS, often within a few days.

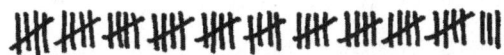

Tape the Reminder Card to your computer. You can also use it as a bookmark. Put it a few pages ahead, and when you reach it, take a break and add a bar to the gate. Then put it a few more pages ahead and continue reading.

Diabetic Retinopathy

Diabetic retinopathy is a serious eye disease that affects people with diabetes. It occurs when high blood sugar levels cause damage to the blood vessels in the retina. Over time, this damage can lead to vision loss if left untreated.

Causes

Diabetic retinopathy is classified into two main stages: nonproliferative diabetic retinopathy (NPDR) and proliferative diabetic retinopathy (PDR). In NPDR, the walls of the blood vessels in the retina weaken, causing tiny bulges called *microaneurysms* to form. These microaneurysms can leak fluid and blood into the retina, leading to swelling and blurred vision. As the condition progresses, blood vessels can become blocked, preventing blood from reaching the retina.

In PDR, the retina grows new, abnormal blood vessels in an attempt to improve blood circulation. These new vessels are fragile and can leak blood into the vitreous, the gel-like substance that fills the eye. This can cause dark floaters, vision loss, and even retinal detachment.

Symptoms

Early stages of diabetic retinopathy may not show any symptoms. However, as the condition progresses, symptoms such as floaters, blurred vision, dark or empty areas in the visual field vision, and poor night vision may appear. It's important to note that diabetic retinopathy usually affects both eyes.

Several factors increase the risk of diabetic retinopathy, including the duration of diabetes, poor blood sugar control, high blood pressure, high cholesterol, obesity, and tobacco use. Pregnant women with diabetes are also at higher risk.

Treatment
Treatment options for diabetic retinopathy depend on the severity of the condition. In the early stages, managing blood sugar levels and blood pressure may be sufficient. For more advanced cases, treatments such as laser surgery, injections of medications into the eye, and surgery to remove the vitreous may be necessary.

Management
Managing diabetes is crucial in preventing diabetic retinopathy. This includes maintaining healthy blood sugar levels, controlling blood pressure, and avoiding tobacco use. Regular eye exams with dilation are essential for early detection and treatment.

Vision Therapy for Diabetic Retinopathy
All vision therapy must be done under the supervision of an eye care professional. Do entended periods of Hydrotherapy and Palming in order to stimulate blood flow to the eyes and facilitate the healing process. Repeat the affirmation "My eyes are getting better and my vision is improving!"

Do not do any of the other exercises. Eat plenty of fruits and vegetables and take a high-quality vitamin supplement such as Bausch & Lomb's PreserVision (AREDS 2), which contains the formula advocated by the National Eye Institute against age-related diseases.

Dry Eye Disease

Dry eye disease (DED) is a common condition that occurs when your eyes don't produce enough tears or the quality of your tears is poor. Tears are essential for keeping the surface of your eyes lubricated, smooth, and clear. When there's a problem with the tear film, it can lead to uncomfortable symptoms such as burning, itching, and a gritty feeling in your eyes.

Causes
Several factors can contribute to dry eye disease, including:

- **Age.** Tear production tends to decrease as we age.

- **Gender.** Women are more likely to develop dry eye, especially after menopause.

- **Medical conditions.** Diseases such as rheumatoid arthritis, Sjögren's syndrome, thyroid disorders, and lupus can cause dry eye.

- **Environmental factors.** Exposure to wind, smoke, and dry air can exacerbate dry eye symptoms.

- **Medications.** Certain medications, including antihistamines, decongestants, and antidepressants, can reduce tear production.

Symptoms

Common symptoms include a stinging, burning, or scratchy sensation in your eyes; mucus in or around your eyes; eye redness; a sensation of having something in your eyes; sensitivity to bright light; difficulty with night-time driving.

Treatment

The goal is to restore the normal amount of tears in the eye to minimize dryness and discomfort. Options include:

- **Artificial tears.** Over-the-counter eye drops that help lubricate the eyes.

- **Prescription eye drops.** Medications that increase tear production or reduce inflammation.

- **Lifestyle changes.** Using a humidifier and taking breaks from screen time can help manage symptoms.

- **Surgical options.** In severe cases, procedures like punctal plugs or special lenses may be recommended.

- **Vision therapy.** Eye exercises can stimulate the production of tear fluid naturally.

What Is Sjögren's Syndrome?

Sjögren's syndrome is a type of dry eye disease caused by an autoimmune disorder affecting the glands that produce tears and saliva, leading to dry eyes and a dry mouth. It can also cause joint pain, fatigue, and dry skin.

Causes

Sjögren's syndrome occurs when the immune system attacks the body's own cells and tissues. The exact cause is unknown but is believed to involve a combination of genetic and environmental factors.

Diagnosis/Treatment

The primary symptoms of Sjögren's syndrome are dry eyes and dry mouth. Other symptoms may include joint pain, swelling, and stiffness; swollen salivary glands; skin rashes or dry skin; persistent dry cough; fatigue.

Treatment

Diagnosing Sjögren's syndrome can be difficult due to its nonspecific symptoms. Tests may include blood tests, eye exams, and imaging studies. Treatment focuses on managing symptoms and preventing complications. This may involve:

- **Artificial tears and saliva substitutes.** To relieve dryness.

- **Medications.** To reduce inflammation and manage pain.

- **Lifestyle changes.** Such as using a humidifier and staying hydrated.

- **Regular dental care.** To prevent tooth decay and other oral health issues that may affect saliva production.

Vision Therapy for Dry Eye Disease

Dry eye disease can often be cured with vision therapy. Do plenty of Squeeze Blinking, Slow Blinking, Hydrotherapy, and Palming. Repeat the affirmation "My eyes are getting better and my vision is improving!"

Floaters

Floaters are small, dark shapes that appear to float in your field of vision. They are often described as structures that look like cobwebs or threads and are most noticeable when looking at a plain, bright background such as the sky or a white wall. Floaters are tiny clumps of dead cells or protein inside the vitreous, the clear substance that fills the eye.

Causes

Floaters are usually caused by age-related changes in the vitreous. As we age, the vitreous shrinks and becomes more liquid. This can cause the vitreous to pull away from the retina. When this happens, it can create clumps of dead cells or protein gel that cast shadows on the retina, which we see as floaters. Other factors that can cause floaters include:

- **Posterior vitreous detachment.** This occurs when the vitreous separates from the retina and is a common cause of floaters in older adults.

- **Eye injuries.** Trauma to the eye can cause bleeding or inflammation, leading to floaters.

- **Eye surgery.** Certain eye surgeries can cause floaters as a side effect.

- **Eye diseases.** Conditions such as retinal detachment can also cause floaters.

Symptoms

Most floaters are harmless and do not require treatment. However, if you notice a sudden increase in floaters, especially if accompanied by flashes of light or a shadow in your peripheral vision, it could indicate a more serious problem like retinal detachment. In such cases, it is important to see an eye care professional immediately.

Treatment

For most people, floaters are a minor annoyance that can be ignored. Eventually, the visual system learns to see around them. However, if floaters significantly interfere with vision, there are treatment options available:

- **Laser therapy.** A laser can be used to break up the floaters, making them less noticeable.

- **Vitrectomy.** This is a surgical procedure where the vitreous gel is removed and replaced with a saline solution. This is usually reserved for severe cases.

Prevention/Management

While there is no guaranteed way to prevent floaters, maintaining overall eye health can help reduce the risk of developing them. This includes:

- **Regular eye exams.** Routine eye exams can help detect any changes in the vitreous or retina early on.

- **Protecting your eyes.** Wearing protective eyewear during sports or activities that could lead to eye injuries can help prevent floaters caused by trauma.

- **Managing chronic conditions.** Keeping conditions like diabetes and high blood pressure under control can reduce the risk of eye complications that may lead to floaters.

Conclusion

Floaters are a common and usually harmless part of aging. Although they can be annoying, they usually do not require treatment. However, if you experience a sudden increase in floaters or other symptoms like flashes of light or a shadow in your vision, it is important to seek medical attention promptly.

Vision Therapy for Floaters

There are no eye exercises effective against floaters.

Glaucoma

Glaucoma is a group of eye diseases that damage the optic nerve, which is crucial for good vision. This damage is often caused by abnormally high pressure in the eye, and can lead to blindness if not treated early. It's often called the *silent thief of sight* because it can progress without noticeable symptoms until significant vision loss has occurred.

Causes

The exact cause of glaucoma is unknown, but several factors increase the risk of developing the disease, including:

- **High eye pressure.** The most common type of glaucoma, primary open-angle glaucoma, is often associated with increased pressure inside the eye.

- **Age.** People over the age of 40 are at higher risk, and the risk increases with age.

- **Family history.** A family history of glaucoma increases the likelihood of developing the condition.

- **Ethnicity.** African Americans over the age of 40 and Hispanics over the age of 60 are at higher risk.

- **Medical conditions.** Conditions like diabetes, high blood pressure, and heart disease can increase the risk.

- **Eye injuries.** Trauma to the eye can lead to secondary glaucoma.

There are two main types of glaucoma:

- **Open-angle glaucoma**. This is the most common form and develops slowly over time without any symptoms. It's often detected during a routine eye exam.

- **Angle-closure glaucoma**. This type occurs suddenly and is a medical emergency. Symptoms may include severe nausea, or pain or redness in the eye, or seeing halos around lights, or blurred vision.

Symptoms

In the early stages, glaucoma usually has no symptoms and vision appears to be normal. As the disease progresses, peripheral vision is usually affected first. If left untreated, glaucoma can lead to significant vision loss and blindness in some cases.

Diagnosis

Early detection is key to preventing vision loss. Regular eye exams are recommended, especially for those at higher risk. During an eye exam, the eye professional will measure the pressure inside your eyes, inspect the drainage angle, examine your optic nerve, and test your peripheral vision.

Treatment

Treatment for glaucoma aims to lower eye pressure to prevent further damage to the optic nerve. Options include:

- **Medications.** Eye drops or oral medications can help reduce eye pressure.

- **Laser therapy.** Laser trabeculoplasty can improve drainage of fluid in the eye.

- **Surgery.** In some cases, surgery may be necessary to create a new drainage path for fluid in the eye.

Management

Although glaucoma cannot be prevented, early detection and treatment can help manage the condition and prevent significant vision loss. Regular eye exams are crucial. Managing underlying health conditions, such as diabetes and high blood pressure, can also help reduce the risk.

Vision Therapy for Glaucoma

All vision therapy must be done under the supervision of an eye care professional. Do Hydrotherapy and Palming for extended periods of time. Do not do any of the other exercises.

Repeat the affirmation "My eyes are getting better and my vision is improving!"

Eat plenty of fruits and vegetables and take a vitamin supplement for the eyes such as Bausch & Lomb's PreserVision (AREDS 2).

Hyperopia (Farsightedness)

Hyperopia, also known as *farsightedness*, is a common visual problem where distant objects can usually be seen clearly, but close objects may appear blurry. This happens because of the shape of the eye, which causes light to focus behind the retina instead of directly on it. Hyperopia is a refractive error. It is not a disease, and it usually occurs in both eyes.

Causes

Hyperopia occurs when the eye is shorter than normal or the cornea does not have enough curvature. As a result, the eye can't properly focus light onto the retina. Genetics often play a significant role, so if either of your parents has hyperopia, you are more likely to have it too.

Prevalence

Almost all babies are born with a slight amount of hyperopia. This usually disappears as the child grows, dropping to 21% of children age 6 months, 8.4% of children age 6 years, 2.5% of children age 12 years, and 1% of children age 15 years.

Consequently, hyperopia is rare among adults. However, many people who previously had good vision lose their ability to focus on near objects around the age of 40 and incorrectly think they are farsighted. In fact, the loss of focusing power in older adults is due to presbyopia (aging eyes), which is a completely different disorder.

Symptoms

Generally, a farsighted person sees distant objects clearly, but near vision is blurry. You may also experience eyestrain, headaches, and difficulty reading or doing other close-up tasks. In children, symptoms may not be noticeable because their eyes are more flexible and often compensate for the issue, but they may squint to see clearly, or struggle with schoolwork, or complain of tired, aching eyes.

Diagnosis

Eye care professionals can diagnose hyperopia through a comprehensive eye exam. They will use various instruments and tests to measure how light enters your eyes and how well you can see at different distances.

With patients who can read the letters on an eye chart, they may use an instrument known as a *phoropter* to determine the refractive error. With young children who cannot read an eye chart, they may use an instrument called a *retinoscope* to see where light is focused inside the eye. If a child fails to outgrow hyperopia, it must be treated or it can lead to a lazy eye or crossed eyes.

Treatment

There are several ways to treat hyperopia. It should be noted that glasses and contact lenses relieve the symptoms but do not correct the underlying problem. Surgery and vision therapy aim to correct the underlying problem:

- **Glasses.** The most common and simplest solution that compensates for the refractive error and allows light to be properly focused onto the retina.

- **Contact lenses.** Another option that provides a wider field of view and is often preferred for aesthetic reasons.

- **Refractive surgery.** Procedures like LASIK or PRK can reshape the cornea to correct the focus.

- **Vision therapy.** In children with abnormal amounts of hyperopia, optometric visual training can usually correct the underlying problem. In hyperopic adults, vision therapy eye exercises can usually increase the eye's natural focusing power to some extent.

Management

While you can't prevent hyperopia, you can manage its symptoms effectively with minimum disruption. Hyperopia is common in young children, but rare in adults. Regular eye exams are crucial, especially for young children, to identify and treat hyperopia early. Maintaining a healthy lifestyle, including a balanced diet rich in vitamins A, C, and E, can keep the eyes healthy and help them grow normally.

Vision Therapy for Hyperopia

Do all the Power Vision Program Exercises with emphasis on Flexing, Pushups, Conducting, and the Fusion Charts. The goal is to increase the flexibility and focusing range of your inner lenses. Work at getting your blur threshold as close to your eyes as possible.

Try to read without glasses or use weaker glasses. Don't use bifocals. Use the Reminder Card as a bookmark. Put it a few pages ahead and practice your New Visual Habits when you reach it. Study the shape of the words and individual letters; then put the Reminder Card a few more pages ahead.

Macular Degeneration

Macular degeneration is a common eye disease that affects the macula, the central part of the retina responsible for sharp, detailed vision. It's a leading cause of vision loss in people over the age of 50 and is usually caused in much the same way as cataracts—poor nutrition and buildup of cellular waste products. There are two main types of macular degeneration: dry (atrophic) and wet (exudative).

Dry Macular Degeneration

This is the more common form, accounting for about 85 to 90% of cases. It occurs when the macula thins over time, leading to a gradual loss of central vision. While there is no cure for dry macular degeneration, certain lifestyle changes and nutritional supplements may slow its progression. These include a diet rich in leafy greens, fish, and nuts, as well as supplements containing vitamins C, E, zinc, and copper.

Wet Macular Degeneration

This is less common but more severe. It occurs when abnormal blood vessels grow under the macula and leak fluid or blood, causing rapid and severe vision loss. Treatment for wet macular degeneration may include intraocular injections of anti-VEGF medications, which can reduce the growth of abnormal blood vessels and slow vision loss.

Several factors can increase the risk of developing macular degeneration, including age, genetics, smoking, and exposure to UV light. Maintaining a healthy lifestyle, including regular exercise and a balanced diet, can reduce the risk.

Symptoms

Early symptoms of macular degeneration may include blurred or distorted vision, difficulty reading, and a dark or empty spot in the center of vision. As the condition progresses, these symptoms may become more pronounced, affecting activities such as driving and recognizing faces.

Diagnosis/Treatment

If you experience any symptoms of macular degeneration, it's important to see an eye care professional for a comprehensive eye examination. Tests such as the Amsler grid can help detect early signs of the condition. Although macular degeneration cannot be cured, early detection and treatment can help manage the disease and improve quality of life.

For those with significant vision loss, vision rehabilitation can be beneficial. This may include low vision devices such as magnifying glasses and telescopic lenses, as well as training to use the person's remaining vision more effectively.

Conclusion

Macular degeneration is a serious eye disease that can significantly impact vision and reduce the quality of life. Understanding the risk factors, symptoms, and treatment options can help individuals take proactive steps to manage the condition and maintain their vision. Regular eye exams and a healthy lifestyle are key to preventing and managing macular degeneration.

Vision Therapy for Macular Degeneration

All vision therapy must be done under the supervision of an eye care professional. Do Hydrotherapy and Palming for extended periods of time in order to stimulate blood flow and nutrition to the eyes. Do not do any other exercises. Repeat the affirmation "My eyes are getting better and my vision is improving!"

Eat plenty of fruits and vegetables and take a high-quality vitamin supplement such as Bausch & Lomb's PreserVision (AREDS 2), which contains the formula advocated by the National Eye Institute against macular degeneration.

Myopia (Nearsightedness)

Myopia, also known as *nearsightedness*, is a common vision problem where distant objects are blurry while close objects can be seen clearly. It affects nearly 30% of the American population and is becoming prevalent worldwide as more people use computers and smartphones.

Causes

Myopia occurs when the eyeball is too long or the cornea is too curved. This causes light entering the eye to focus incorrectly, resulting in blurred distance vision. Myopia is a refractive error and usually affects both eyes. It is not a disease, although progressive myopia can lead to potentially blinding diseases such as glaucoma and retinal detachment. Several factors contribute to the development of myopia:

- **Genetics.** Myopia often runs in families. If one or both parents are nearsighted, there is a higher chance their children will also develop myopia.

- **Environmental factors.** Spending long periods doing close-up work, such as reading, using computers, or playing video games, is the primary cause of myopia.

- **Night myopia.** Some people experience blurred distance vision only at night due to low light conditions, which make it difficult for the eyes to focus properly.

- **Pseudo myopia.** This occurs when the eyes become temporarily fatigued from prolonged close-up work, causing blurred distance vision.

- **Corrective lenses.** Doing close work through glasses or contact lenses that were prescribed for distance vision usually causes myopia to get worse.

Symptoms

People with myopia usually experience difficulty seeing far objects clearly such as road signs, a whiteboard in school, or a movie screen, often accompanied by eyestrain or headaches from squinting to see better.

Diagnosis

Eye care professionals can diagnose myopia by means of a comprehensive eye exam, which includes tests to measure how the eyes focus light and determine the power of any optical lenses needed to compensate for the refractive error. The most common test is the visual acuity test, where you identify letters on a chart 20 feet away.

Treatment

The traditional method of treating myopia is to prescribe glasses or contact lenses that compensate for the refractive error (corrective lenses). Special lenses such as low plus or bifocals are often used to reduce visual stress from close activities and slow myopic progression. Vision therapy can also be beneficial.

For adults, laser and other surgical procedures are available to reduce or eliminate reliance on glasses or contact lenses. Good visual habits, such as taking frequent breaks during close work and proper lighting, can help prevent or reduce myopic progression, especially in children and young adults.

Prevention

Although genetics can play a significant role in the development of myopia, adopting good visual habits can prevent myopia or slow its progression. Encouraging children to spend more time outdoors and maintain proper posture while reading, as well as ensuring adequate lighting, can make a difference.

Conclusion

Myopia is a common vision problem that can significantly impact a person's life. Understanding its causes, symptoms, and management is crucial for maintaining good eye health. Getting regular eye exams and adopting healthy visual habits can help prevent or manage myopia effectively.

Vision Therapy for Myopia

We have found that incipient and low myopia are often easy to reverse with vision therapy eye exercises, allowing return to normal or near-normal vision. High myopia can show significant improvement, often resulting in a weaker prescription as the deterioration is reversed.

Do all the exercises in all the modules with emphasis on Flexing, Pushups, Blinking, Clocking, Detailing, the Biofeedback Charts, and the Fusion Charts. The goal is to increase the focusing range and flexibility of the inner lens.

In addition, use the following strategy when doing close work. Instead of reading page after page without stopping or spending hour after hour gazing at a computer screen, take frequent breaks. Close your eyes for a few seconds; then open them and look at a far object or something across the room. Do plenty of blinking to keep your eyes moist and lubricated.

Discipline yourself to take 50 breaks per day and keep a written record using *bars and gates*. Every time you take a break, add a bar to the gate. This simple strategy prevents nearpoint stress from building up, which is the major cause of myopia.

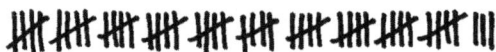

Tape the Reminder Card to your computer. You can also use it as a bookmark. Put it a few pages ahead, and when you reach it, take a break and add a bar to the gate. Then put it a few more pages ahead and continue reading.

Spend more time outdoors, especially in natural surroundings. Gaze at distant objects and take in as much space as possible.

How to Use Glasses

It's important not to wear distance glasses or contacts for long periods of reading or computer work, because they usually cause the myopia to get worse! If you can't read without them, use the weakest prescription that gives you good vision at your normal reading distance but makes everything farther away blurred.

Many people have old weaker glasses that will suffice. If you don't have any, ask your optometrist to prescribe weaker glasses for reading and computer work. This strategy works best for people with less than −3.0D of myopia.

If you have a small amount of myopia, you may be able to use stress relieving lenses. If your work requires you to look up frequently and see far objects clearly, ask your optometrist to prescribe bifocals using Professor Young's formula (see Section 9).

Pink Eye (Conjunctivitis)

Pink eye, also known as *conjunctivitis*, is a common eye disease that causes inflammation of the conjunctiva, the thin membrane that covers the white part of the eye and the inner surface of the eyelids. This inflammation makes the blood vessels in the conjunctiva more visible, giving the eye a pink or red appearance.

Causes

Pink eye can be caused by several factors, including:

- **Viral infections.** The most common cause, often associated with the same viruses that cause the common cold.

- **Bacterial infections.** Caused by bacteria such as *Staphylococcus aureus* and *Streptococcus pneumoniae*.

- **Allergic reactions.** Triggered by allergens like pollen, dust, and pet dander.

- **Irritants.** Such as smoke, chlorine in swimming pools, and shampoos.

- **Contact lenses.** Improper use or hygiene of contact lenses can also lead to pink eye.

Viral and bacterial forms of pink eye are highly contagious through contact with an infected person's eye secretions or by touching surfaces contaminated with these secretions. Sharing personal items like towels, makeup, and contact lenses can also spread the infection.

Symptoms

The symptoms of pink eye can vary depending on the cause but often include redness in one or both eyes, itchiness and a gritty feeling in the eyes, watery discharge, crusting of the eyelids, sensitivity to bright light.

Diagnosis/Treatment

Diagnosis is usually based on symptoms and a physical examination of the eye. In some cases, a sample of the discharge may be taken for testing to determine the exact cause. Treatment depends on the cause:

- **Viral conjunctivitis.** There is no specific treatment; it usually resolves on its own within one to two weeks. Cool compresses and artificial tears can help relieve symptoms.

- **Bacterial conjunctivitis.** Antibiotic eye drops or ointments are prescribed to treat the infection.

- **Allergic conjunctivitis.** Avoiding allergens and using antihistamine eye drops can help reduce symptoms.

- **Irritant conjunctivitis.** Removing the irritant and using lubricating eye drops can provide relief.

Prevention

Pink eye can be prevented *with* good hygiene:

- **Wash hands frequently** with soap and water.

- **Avoid touching the eyes**, especially with unwashed hands.

- **Do not share personal items** like towels, makeup, and contact lenses.

- **Clean surfaces** that may be contaminated with eye secretions.

Complications

While pink eye is usually a mild condition, complications can occur, especially if left untreated. These may include:

- **Corneal inflammation** (keratitis)

- **Blepharitis** (inflammation of the eyelids)

- **Vision loss** in severe cases

Vision Therapy for Pink Eye

There are no eye exercises that are effective against pink eye. Palming and Hydrotherapy may relieve the discomfort and encourage the eyes to heal. Repeat the affirmation "My eyes are getting better and my vision is improving!"

Presbyopia (Aging Eyes)

Presbyopia is a common visual problem that affects almost everyone as they grow older. It typically becomes noticeable in the mid-40s and is characterized by difficulty focusing on close objects. Presbyopia is a refractive error. It is often combined with existing refractive errors such as myopia or astigmatism, and is often confused with hyperopia (farsightedness). It is not a disease.

Causes

As we age, the eye's inner lens becomes less flexible. This loss of flexibility makes it harder for the inner lens to change shape and focus light directly onto the retina, which is necessary for clear vision. This results in blurred vision when looking at close objects.

Symptoms

Common symptoms include difficulty seeing objects up close, blurred vision at normal reading distance, the need to hold reading material at arm's length to see it clearly, eyestrain and headaches when doing close work.

Diagnosis/Treatment

A comprehensive eye exam will determine if you have presbyopia. An eye care professional will measure your near and far vision and will determine the appropriate measures. Treatment options for presbyopia include:

- **Reading glasses.** These are designed to help with close-up vision and can be purchased from drugstores and other stores without a prescription, although it's best to get an eye exam to determine the correct power.

- **Bifocals, trifocals, or progressive lenses.** These glasses have multiple lens areas to improve vision at different distances.

- **Contact lenses.** Monovision contact lenses improve one eye for distance vision and the other for close-up vision, while multifocal lenses have different powers for near and far vision.

- **Surgical options.** Procedures like LASIK and lens implants can also improve presbyopia.

- **Vision therapy.** Eye exercises can often reverse or delay presbyopia by improving the flexibility of the eye's inner lens.

Conclusion

Presbyopia is a natural part of the aging process and cannot be prevented, although it can often be reversed or delayed with vision therapy. By understanding its causes, symptoms, and treatment options, individuals can take steps to maintain clear and comfortable vision.

Vision Therapy for Presbyopia

The fluids inside the eye circulate as a result of the ciliary muscle and the iris sphincter muscle expanding and contracting and the inner lens changing its shape.

Nutrients are pumped into the eye from the posterior base of the ciliary muscle, and cellular waste products are pumped out of the eye through Schlemm's canal, which is located at the anterior base of the iris sphincter muscle.

As we get older, the inner lens loses its flexibility. Nutrients can't get in, and waste products can't get out. The inner lens is starved of nutrition, and waste products clog the tiny exit channels. This makes the problem worse and reduces the flexibility of the inner lens even further.

Vision therapy for presbyopia is concerned with maximizing the activity of the ciliary muscle and the iris sphincter muscle and the flexibility of the inner lens. The goal is to increase the nutrient flow to the inner lens and the exodus of waste products. This makes the eyes healthier and helps them function properly.

Do all the exercises in all the modules with emphasis on Flexing, Pushups, Conducting, and the Fusion Charts. Work at getting your blur threshold as close to your eyes as possible.

Try to read without glasses or use weaker glasses. Don't use bifocals. Use the Reminder Card as a bookmark. Put it a few pages ahead and practice your New Visual Habits when you reach it. Study the shape of the words and individual letters; then put the Reminder Card a few more pages ahead.

Retinal Detachment

Retinal detachment is a serious condition that occurs when the retina pulls away from its normal position on the inside of the eyeball. This can lead to permanent vision loss if not treated promptly.

Causes

There are three main types of retinal detachment: rhegmatogenous, tractional, and exudative.

- **Rhegmatogenous retinal detachment.** This is the most common type and usually occurs due to a tear or hole in the retina. The vitreous gel inside the eye can seep through the tear and accumulate behind the retina, causing it to detach. Risk factors for rhegmatogenous retinal detachment include aging, severe nearsightedness, eye injuries, and previous eye surgeries.

- **Tractional retinal detachment.** This occurs when scar tissue on the retina's surface contracts and pulls the retina away from its underlying tissue. This type is often associated with conditions like diabetic retinopathy, where damaged blood vessels can lead to the formation of scar tissue.

- **Exudative retinal detachment.** This is a condition where fluid accumulates behind the retina without the presence of a tear. This can happen due to inflammation, injury, or other conditions that cause fluid leakage behind the retina.

Symptoms

These may include the sudden appearance of floaters, flashes of light, blurred vision, and a shadow or curtain effect over part of the visual field. These symptoms require immediate medical attention to prevent permanent vision loss.

Several factors increase the risk of retinal detachment, including aging, high myopia, eye injuries, previous eye surgeries, and a family history of retinal detachment.

Diagnosis

Diagnosing retinal detachment involves a comprehensive eye examination, including dilation of the pupil to allow a detailed view of the retina. Imaging tests such as ultrasound may also be used to confirm the diagnosis.

Treatment

Treatment typically involves surgery to reattach the retina. Common surgical procedures include laser photocoagulation, cryopexy (freezing), and pneumatic retinopexy (injecting a gas bubble into the eye to push the retina back into place). In more severe cases, a vitrectomy (removal of the vitreous gel) may be necessary.

Prevention

Although some risk factors cannot be changed, maintaining a healthy lifestyle and protecting the eyes from injury can help reduce the risk. Regular eye exams are crucial for early detection and timely treatment.

For individuals who experience vision loss due to retinal detachment, vision rehabilitation can be beneficial. This may include low vision aids, such as magnifying glasses and telescopic lenses, as well as training to use the remaining vision more effectively.

Conclusion

Retinal detachment is a serious condition that requires immediate medical attention to prevent permanent vision loss. Understanding the risk factors, symptoms, and treatment options can help individuals take proactive steps to protect their vision. Regular eye exams and prompt treatment are key to managing retinal detachment and maintaining eye health.

Vision Therapy for Retinal Detachment

All vision therapy must be done under the supervision of an eye care professional. Do extended periods of Hydrotherapy and Palming in order to stimulate blood flow and facilitate the healing process. Do not do any of the other exercises. Repeat the affirmation "My eyes are getting better and my vision is improving!"

Eat plenty of fruits and vegetables and take a high-quality vitamin supplement such as Bausch & Lomb's PreserVision (AREDS 2), which contains the formula advocated by the National Eye Institute against age-related diseases.

Strabismus (Crossed Eyes)

Commonly known as *crossed eyes*, strabismus is a condition where the eyes do not align properly. This misalignment can cause one eye to turn inward, outward, upward, or downward. Strabismus can affect children and adults, so understanding it is crucial for effective management and treatment.

Occurrence

Strabismus occurs when the extraocular muscles do not work together properly. These muscles receive signals from the brain to coordinate and direct their movements, but if there's a problem with these signals, the eyes may point in different directions. This can happen all the time, or only if a person is stressed, is tired, or has done a lot of close work.

Causes

Several factors can contribute to the development of strabismus, including:

- **Genetics**. A family history of strabismus increases the likelihood of developing the condition.

- **Refractive errors**. Hyperopia (farsightedness) can lead to strabismus because the eyes must work harder to focus.

- **General health conditions**. Conditions like Down syndrome, cerebral palsy, and brain injuries can also cause strabismus.

- **Eye injuries**. Trauma to the eye or surrounding structures can result in strabismus.

Symptoms

Common symptoms include:

- **Misaligned eyes.** One eye may turn inward (esotropia), outward (exotropia), upward (hypertropia), or downward (hypotropia). In many cases, the misalignment may not be noticeable and one eye may seem to be slightly "off."

- **Double vision.** When the eyes are misaligned, the brain receives two different images, leading to double vision.

- **Squinting or frequent blinking.** People with strabismus may squint or blink frequently, especially in bright light.

- **Head tilting.** To align their vision, individuals may tilt their head to one side.

- **Poor depth perception.** Misaligned eyes can affect depth perception, making it difficult to judge distances.

- **Eyestrain and headaches.** Strabismus can cause eye strain and headaches due to the extra effort needed to focus.

Diagnosis/Treatment

Diagnosing strabismus involves a comprehensive eye exam, including a refraction test to determine the prescription of glasses and an evaluation of eye alignment. Treatment options depend on the severity and type of strabismus and may include:

- **Glasses or contact lenses.** These can compensate for refractive errors that may be contributing to strabismus.

- **Prism lenses.** Prisms can be added to glasses to help align the eyes.

- **Vision therapy.** This is a structured program of visual activities designed to improve eye coordination and alignment. Vision therapy is often used in conjunction with other treatments.

- **Surgery.** In some cases, surgery may be necessary to adjust the muscles controlling eye movement. Vision therapy may be recommended before and after surgery to stabilize eye alignment.

- **Botox.** Injections of Botox temporarily weaken the muscles responsible for the misalignment and are a common alternative to surgery.

Conclusion

Living with strabismus can be challenging, but with proper treatment and care, most individuals can lead a normal life. It's essential to work closely with an eye care professional to develop a personalized treatment plan.

Vision Therapy for Strabismus

Many traditional eye doctors, especially ophthalmologists, believe that strabismus is a genetic defect. They have been taught that one of the extraocular muscles is attached to the wrong position on the eyeball, causing the eye to point in the wrong direction.

They treat strabismus by surgically attaching the "bad" eye muscle to a new position. Unfortunately, strabismus surgery is not very effective, with a success rate of only 20%. In most cases, the eyes remain straight for a few months, then become crossed again and need additional surgeries.

Modern advances in vision care have made strabismus surgery obsolete. It should not be used unless all other methods have failed. Botox and vision therapy are much more effective. The Botox is injected into the extraocular muscles to straighten the eyes, which usually remain straight when the drug eventually wears off. This should be accompanied by vision therapy to make the eyes work together as a team. Do all the eye exercises in the Power Vision Program.

SECTION

9

PRESCRIBING GUIDE FOR EYE CARE PROFESSIONALS

The Power Vision Program provides health-conscious doctors and their patients with a therapeutic method of treating common visual problems such as amblyopia, asthenopia, astigmatism, computer vision syndrome, hyperopia, myopia, and presbyopia. Therapeutic guidelines are also provided for patients with cataracts, macular degeneration, and retinal detachment.

The techniques reliably improve acuity, usually with a significant reduction of refractive error. However, the reduction of refractive error is not enough to account for the magnitude of acuity improvement, and we have identified nine different acuity improvement mechanisms that are outlined at the end of this section.

The Power Vision Program emphasizes acuity improvement with little or no attempt to develop other visual skills. This significantly reduces the time needed to get results, and most patients feel positive changes in their eyes and see an improvement in acuity within a week or so. The Power Vision Program is designed to help the following groups of patients:

Group One: Patients with incipient or minor visual problems, such as asthenopia in emmetropia, low myopia, computer vision syndrome, low hyperopia, low astigmatism, or early presbyopia, can often avoid, delay, or eliminate the need for corrective lenses. Good results are usually obtained within a month. Asthenopia caused by reading or computer work is surprisingly easy to treat, and most patients report a major reduction in discomfort within a few days.

Group Two: Patients with unstable visual problems, such as medium to high astigmatism, hyperopia, myopia, or presbyopia, can usually stabilize their condition and prevent or delay further deterioration, thereby avoiding or delaying the need for a stronger prescription. Stabilization can usually be achieved within a few weeks.

Group Three: Highly motivated patients with stable visual problems, such as medium to high astigmatism, hyperopia, myopia, or presbyopia, can usually adapt to a series of progressively weaker corrective lenses and eliminate or reduce their dependency on them. Several months of therapy are usually needed to obtain maximum results.

The Power Vision Program does not promise a return to emmetropia. Although this happens in many cases, most patients with large refractive errors must do the exercises for several months before they achieve a major improvement, and they usually deem this to be a worthwhile investment in their health-oriented lifestyle.

The Power Vision Program provides you with a professionally designed method of helping health-conscious patients, enabling them to play an active role in their vision care. It is not a "throw away your glasses" gimmick. It is based on well-established principles of behavioral optometry with an emphasis on improving ocular health and visual acuity together with other visual skills if necessary. For the sake of simplicity, we use *eyesight* and *vision* interchangeably throughout the Power Vision Program, although these terms have rather different meanings.

Mydriatic or cycloplegic examinations should only be performed after functional testing, or on a different day. These drugs create spherical and chromatic aberrations that are not part of the patient's usual visual performance and complicate retinoscopy and subjective testing. These drugs also diminish diagnostic capability by preventing the evaluation of accommodation and the accommodative convergence function.

Therapeutic Lens Prescribing

Group One: Patients with incipient visual problems should not be corrected for refractive error. Patients with minor visual problems should receive an undercorrection that gives 20/40 binocular acuity at the distance for which the lenses are normally used. Ignore astigmatism up to 1.00D.

Group Two: Since the goal is to reverse deterioration and stabilize vision through the current prescription, additional lenses are usually not needed.

Group Three: Undercorrect to 20/40 binocular acuity at the distance for which the lenses are normally used. Myopes should receive a 20/40 undercorrection for driving. Myopes who engage in close work should receive a separate prescription that undercorrects to 20/40 binocular acuity at the working distance. Hyperopes and presbyopes should be undercorrected for reading and close work. Ignore astigmatism up to 1.00D depending on the axis, but undercorrect larger amounts by one-third. If bifocals are needed, undercorrect both segments.

Continue to periodically reduce the strength of the lenses until the patient achieves the maximum amount of improvement. This strategy is known as *progressive undercorrection*. Patients who use disposable contacts should receive a series of lenses with 0.25D decrements.

Stress-Relieving Lenses

Patients with asthenopia, computer vision syndrome, and incipient or low myopia who engage in long periods of close work should receive stress-relieving lenses to prevent or reduce the amount of accommodation. These lenses should contain the maximum amount of plus that is acceptable at the normal working distance. Stress-relieving lenses enable the eyes to perform the nearpoint task as if they are looking at a distant object, thereby avoiding nearpoint stress. Base-in prism may be used to prevent convergence.

Many behavioral optometrists prescribe +0.50D lenses. Although these lenses can reduce physiological stress, they don't completely prevent accommodation and it may be better to use more plus, depending on the patient's ability to accept it. It may also be helpful to prescribe glasses for TV viewing with the maximum amount of plus that will give satisfactory acuity at a distance of 10 to 12 feet. The goal of these lenses is not stress reduction but plus acceptance to reduce accommodation and esophoria.

Young's Formula

The treatment of myopia deserves special consideration. Young's research with illiterate Inuits, identical twins, and captive monkeys clearly shows that myopia is usually the result of sustained focusing on near objects. This creates nearpoint stress, which increases the intraocular pressure (IOP) and causes the eyeball to gradually elongate. Progressive myopia is usually caused by doing close work through distance lenses, which perpetuate the nearpoint stress and aggravate the problem.

The clinical findings of Oakley and Young deserve special consideration. In a well-designed study involving 418 patients, bifocals reduced the average annual rate of myopic progression from −0.52D to −0.02D. The prescription is especially useful for schoolchildren who may not be able to follow a course of vision therapy.

The upper lens is for distance vision such as looking at a whiteboard and is undercorrected by 0.5D. The lower lens is for reading and is +2.0D more than the upper lens. For example, a −4.00D myope will receive a −3.50D upper lens together with a −1.50D lower segment; a −1.25D myope will receive a −0.75D upper lens together with a +1.25D lower segment.

The position of the lower segment is of critical importance. The upper edge must reach the lower edge of the pupil, and the patient should be instructed to use the lower segment for all reading and close work. If the lower segment is below this level, the patient may read through the upper segment and the results will not be as good.

Patient Management

We recommend that you briefly review the Power Vision Program with patients after the initial eye exam and direct them to the appropriate exercises. Then carry out one or more follow-up meetings to encourage compliance, measure acuity, go over the exercises in more detail, and clarify any issues that may arise.

We also recommend holding weekly seminars of patients with similar visual problems, such as a myopia support group or a presbyopia support group. In these seminars, patients can do specific exercises together and discuss areas of improvement and any issues that may arise. Weekly seminars can be very rewarding because they allow you to maintain good contact with patients, who are motivated and encouraged by other patients and the extra care and attention you provide.

An added benefit of weekly seminars is that they can provide an interesting and enjoyable social event where patients mingle with other patients with similar interests and visual problems, often forming new friendships and professional contacts. You can use weekly seminars as a

The Power Vision Program can give you a competitive advantage over optometrists who merely prescribe corrective lenses.

platform for encouraging referrals, handing out promotional materials, and expanding your practice.

The Power Vision Program can give you a competitive advantage over optometrists who merely prescribe corrective lenses. It is professionally gratifying to have patients who are getting better, not worse, and to share their joy and excitement as their condition improves, especially if they are experiencing "flashes" of clear vision.

Doctors who cure or improve their patients' problems will always win gratitude and respect. The sense of satisfaction and personal accomplishment that comes from naturally improved vision is why so many patients refer their friends and relatives. For this reason, behavioral optometrists who provide vision therapy invariably build large, thriving practices.

We therefore invite you to add the Power Vision Program to your arsenal of treatment procedures. To avoid copyright infringement, patients should receive their own copy of the Power Vision Program instead of photocopied material. The Power Vision Program is available at a discount from Humanix Books at (*info@humanixbooks.com*). Local bookstores may also offer bulk discounts.

Acuity Improvement Mechanisms

The techniques used in the Power Vision Program can reduce refractive error, but not enough to account for observed improvements in acuity. We therefore propose the following nine acuity improvement mechanisms. These operate synergistically and can lead to major improvements in acuity—clear flashes—and other visual functions such as fixation, accommodation, and convergence.

Hyperacuity

Even in emmetropia, lenticular and corneal spherical and chromatic aberrations together with diffraction and scattering of light on the retina prevent the formation of a point image. These factors limit the minimum angle of resolution to about 30 arcseconds.

In order to distinguish two-point objects, three bits of information are required: the light from each point object and the absence of light between them. Hence the neural threshold at the fovea requires three cones. The first point object stimulates the first cone, the second cone remains unstimulated, and the second point object stimulates the third cone. For this reason, the neural threshold equals the cone spacing at the fovea, which is about 30 arcseconds.

However, the visual system can resolve differences that are an order of magnitude smaller than the minimum angle of resolution on the retina. For example, it is usually possible to detect a 6-arcsecond difference in the separation of two lines, a 2- to 4-arcsecond vernier displacement, and a 2- to 4-arcsecond separation of lines in a stereoacuity task.

This phenomenon is known as *hyperacuity*. The general principle is that the edge of an object is made to partially overlap cone apertures and hence partially stimulate the cones. If the partial stimulation is sufficient to make the cones fire, the resulting signal can distinguish the position of the object.

We have concluded that ocular microtremors and very small saccades provide the switching mechanism for cone activation. The result is an increase in the signal-to-noise ratio of the retinal data available for image processing by the visual cortex. This mechanism provides a simple explanation of improvements in acuity resulting from edge discrimination training.

Perceptual Enhancement

This is a cerebral acuity improvement mechanism and involves a learning process whereby the edges and textures of blurred objects are enhanced by means of averaging or interpolating the visual data to increase the signal-to-noise ratio, which achieves greater contrast. Perceptual enhancement seems to be an act of selective attention, the visual equivalent of isolating a particular person's voice from the background noise in a room full of chatter.

Ciliary Muscle Tonicity

Ciliary muscle tonicity determines the resting state of the lens in the absence of visual stimulation. Exercising the ciliary muscle will modify its tonicity, thereby changing the resting state of the lens. This is an adaptive change that will extend the nearpoint and farpoint and change the refractive status of the lens.

Extraocular Muscle Tonicity

It is often observed that astigmatism spontaneously changes its magnitude and direction. In most cases, this phenomenon seems to be caused by imbalances in the forces exerted by the extraocular muscles on the eyeball, causing it to change shape. It follows that correcting imbalances will modify extraocular muscle tonicity and change the shape and refractive status of the eyeball.

Accommodative Amplitude

With normal use, the ciliary muscle does not dilate or constrict to its maximum limits. This is especially true of city dwellers, who typically live and work in a confined visual space. It follows that exercising the ciliary muscle will increase the accommodative amplitude, extend the nearpoint and farpoint, and change the refractive status of the lens.

Lenticular Flexibility

It is well established that presbyopia is due to lenticular sclerosis. In view of the fact that physical exercises increase the flexibility of the joints, it follows that eye exercises will increase the flexibility of the lens, thereby modifying its refractive status.

Fixation Disparity

A blurred binocular image cannot be precisely fixated and can lead to convergence errors and diplopia. Since reflex accommodation is largely determined by convergence, fixation disparity may also cause additional loss of focus and acuity. It follows that improving extraocular muscle coordination will refine convergence, reduce fixation disparity, and enable the eyes to focus more accurately with better acuity.

Tear Fluid Contact Lens

Clinical observations show that the stimulation of blinking can cover the cornea with a copious amount of tear fluid, which may form a transient contact lens due to the meniscus curvature at the eyelids, thereby changing the refractive power of the cornea.

Intraocular Pressure

Many myopes and some presbyopes have elevated IOP that seems to be caused by the lens bulging against the iris, which restricts the flow of liquid into the anterior chamber and in some cases impedes drainage through Schlemm's canal. Underlying factors may include chronic nearpoint accommodation in myopes, lenticular growth in presbyopes, and excess sugar consumption.

Our research suggests that excessive IOP can elongate the eyeball and increase myopia. It follows that reducing nearpoint stress and correcting dietary imbalances may reduce the IOP and modify the shape and refractive power of the lens and eyeball.

REFERENCES

Adler-Grinberg D., Questioning our classical understanding of accommodation and presbyopia. *Am. J. Optom. Physiol. Opt.,* 1986, 63(7): 571–580.

Aronsfeld G.H., Eyesight training and development. *J. Am. Optom. Assoc.,* 1936, 7(4): 36–38.

Atkinson, R.P., Sewell, M.M., Enhancement of visual perception under conditions of short-term exposure to sensory isolation. *Percep. Motor Skills,* 1988, 67: 248–252.

Balliet R., Clay A., Blood K., The training of visual acuity in myopia. *J. Am. Optom. Assoc.,* 1982, 53(9): 719–724.

Barber T.X., Changing "unchangeable" bodily processes by suggestions. *Advances,* 1984, 1(2): 7–40.

Beach S.J., Myopia cures. *Trans. Am. Ophth. Soc.,* 1948, 46: 284–294.

Berens C., Girard L.J., Fonda G., Sells S.B., Effects of tachistoscopic training on visual functions in myopic patients. *Am. J. Ophth.,* 1957, 44(3): 1–48.

Beresford S.M., Muris D.W., Allen M.J., Young F.A., Tableman M., Clinical Evaluation of the Power Vision Program. *General Science Journal,* 2021: 8995.

Berman P.E., Levinger S., Massoth N.A., Gallagher D., Kalmar K., Pos L., The effectiveness of biofeedback visual training as a viable method of treatment and reduction of myopia. *J. Optom. Vis. Dev.,* 1985, 16:17–21.

Bettman J.W., Apparent accommodation in aphakic eyes. *Am. J. Ophth.,* 1950, 33(1): 921–928.

Birnbaum M.H., Clinical management of myopia. *Am. J. Optom. Physiol. Opt.,* 1981, 58(7): 554–559.

Ciuffreda K.J., Dynamics of voluntary accommodation. *Am. J. Optom. Physiol. Opt.,* 1988, 65(5): 265–270.

Collins F.L., Epstein L.H., Hannay H.J., A component analysis of an operant training program for improving visual acuity in myopic students. *Behav. Ther.,* 1981, 12: 692–701.

Collins F.L., Ricci J.A., Burkett P.A., Behavioral training for myopia: long term maintenance of improved acuity. *Behav. Res. Ther.,* 1981, 19: 265–268.

Copeland V.L., Increased visual acuity of myopes while in hypnosis. *J. Am. Optom. Assoc.,* 1967, 38(8): 663–664.

Davison G.C., Singleton L., A preliminary report of improved vision under hypnosis. *Int. J. Clin. Exp. Hyp.,* 1967, 15: 57–62.

Epstein L.H., Collins F.L., Hannay H.J., Looney R.L., Fading and feedback in the modification of visual acuity. *J. Behav. Med.,* 1978, 1: 273–297.

Epstein L.H., Greenwald D.J., Monocular feedback and fading training. *Behav. Mod.,* 1981, 5: 171–186.

Eskridge J.B., Review of ciliary muscle effort in presbyopia. *Am. J. Optom. Physiol. Opt.,* 1984, 61(2): 133–138.

Ewalt H., The Baltimore myopia control project. *J. Am. Optom. Assoc.,* 1946, 17(6): 167–185.

Ewalt H.W., Visual training and the presbyopic patient. *J. Am. Optom. Assoc.,* 1959, 30(11): 295–298.

Feldman J., Behavior modification in vision training. *J. Am. Optom. Assoc.,* 1981, 52(4): 329–340.

Forrest E., Eye scan therapy for astigmatism. *J. Am. Optom. Assoc.,* 1984, 55(12): 894–901.

Friedman E., Vision training program for myopia management. *Am. J. Optom. Physiol. Opt.,* 1981, 58(7): 546–553.

Gallop S., Myopia reduction: a view from the inside. *J. Behav. Optom.,* 1994, 5(5): 115–120.

Geisler W.S., Physical limits of acuity and hyperacuity. *J. Opt. Soc. Am.,* 1984, 1(7): 775–782.

Giddings J.W., Lanyon R.I., Effects of reinforcement on visual acuity in myopic adults. *Am. J. Optom. Arch. Am. Acad. Optom.*, 1974, 51(3): 181–188.

Giddings J.W., Lanyon R.I., Modification of refractive error through conditioning. *Behav. Ther.*, 1971, 2(4): 538–542.

Gil K.M., Collins F.L., Behavioral training for myopia. *Behav. Res. Ther.*, 1983, 21(3): 269–273.

Gottlieb R.L., Neuropsychology of myopia. *J. Optom. Vis. Dev.*, 1982, 13(1): 3–27.

Graham C., Leibowitz H.W., The effect of suggestion on visual acuity. *Int. J. Clin. Exp. Hyp.*, 1972, 20(3): 169–186.

Granger L., LeTourneau J., Behavior modification techniques in vision training. *Optom. Wkly.*, 1977, 68(15): 423–427.

Gregg J.R., Variable acuity. *J. Am. Optom. Assoc.*, 1947, 18(3): 432–435.

Hackman R.B., An evaluation of the Baltimore myopia project. *J. Am. Optom. Assoc.*, 1947, 18(4): 416–426.

Hildreth H.R., Mainberg W.H., Milder B., Post L.T., Sanders T.E., The effects of visual training on existing myopia. *Am. J. Ophth.*, 1947, 30: 1563–1576.

Hirsch M.J., Apparent accommodation in aphakia. *Am. J. Optom. Arch. Am. Acad. Optom.*, 1950, 27(8): 412–414.

Hirsch M.J., Prevention and/or cure of myopia. *Am. J. Optom. Arch. Am. Acad. Optom.*, 1965, 42(6): 327–336.

Jensen H., Myopia progression in young schoolchildren and intraocular pressure. *Documenta Ophthalmologica*, 1992, 82(3): 249–255.

Kaplan R., Hypnosis, new horizons for optometry. *Rev. Optom.*, 1978, 115(10): 53–58.

Kelley C.R., Psychological factors in myopia. *J. Am Optom. Assoc.*, 1962, 33(6): 833–837.

Lancaster W.B., Present status of eye exercises. *Arch. Ophth.*, 1944, 32(3): 167–172.

Lancaster W.B., Woods A.C., Hildreth H.R., Visual training for myopia. *J. Am. Med. Assoc.*, 1948, 136: 110.

Lane B., Nutrition and Vision, *J. Optom. Vis. Dev.* 11(3): 1–11, 1980.

Leber L., Wilson T., Myopia reduction training. *J. Behav. Optom.*, 1994, 4(4): 87–92.

References

Le Grande Y., The presence of negative accommodation in certain subjects. *Am. J. Optom. Arch. Am. Acad. Optom.*, 1952, 29: 134–136.

Letourneau J.E., Application of biofeedback and behavior modification techniques in visual training. *J. Optom. Physiol. Opt.*, 1976, 53(4): 187–189.

Levine S.M., Adult visual system plasticity. *J. Am. Optom. Assoc.*, 1988, 59: 135–139.

Marg E., Flashes of clear vision and negative accommodation with reference to the Bates method of visual training. *Am. J. Optom. Arch. Am. Acad. Optom.*, 1952, 29(4): 167–184.

Marg E. An investigation of voluntary as distinguished from reflex accommodation. *Am. J. Optom. Arch. Am. Acad. Optom.*, 1951, 28: 347–356.

National Eye Institute, *Vision Research: A National Plan,* 1999, pp. 100, 102.

Nolan J.A., An approach to myopia control. *Optom. Wkly.*, 1974, 65(6): 149–154.

Oakley K.H., Young F.A., Bifocal control of myopia. *Am J. Optom. Physiol. Opt.*, 1975, 52: 758–764.

Orfield, A., Seeing space: undergoing brain re-programming to reduce myopia. *J. Behav. Optom.*, 1994, 5(5): 123–131.

Pascal J.I., Visual exercises in ophthalmology, *Arch. Ophth.*, 1945, 33: 478.

Poggio, T., Fahle M., Edelman S., Fast perceptual learning in visual hyperacuity. *Science,* 1992, 256: 1018–1021.

Provine R.R., On voluntary ocular accommodation. *Percep. Psychophysics,* 1975, 17(2): 209–212.

Quinn G., Berlin J., Young T., Ziylan S., Stone R., Association of intraocular pressure and myopia in children. *Ophthalmology,* 1992, 102(2): 180–185.

Roscoe S.N., Couchman D.H., Improving visual performance through volitional focus control. *Human Factors,* 1987, 29:311–325.

Sells S.B., Fixott R.S., Evaluation of research on effects of visual training on visual functions. *Am. J. Ophth.,* 1957, 44(2): 230–236.

Sheehan E.P., Smith H.V., Forest D.W., A signal detection study of the effects of suggested improvement on the monocular visual acuity of myopes. *Int. J. Clin. Exp. Hyp.,* 1982, 30: 138–146.

Shepard C.J., The Baltimore project. *Optom. Wkly.,* 1946, 37(5): 133–135.

Sherman A., Myopia can often be prevented, controlled or eliminated. *J. Behav. Optom.,* 1994, 4(1): 16–22.

Sloane A.E., Dunphy E.B., Emmons W.V., The effects of a simple group training method for myopia and visual acuity. *Res. Quart. Am. Assoc. Health,* 1948, 19: 111–117.

Smith E.L., Spectacle lenses and emmetropization. *Optom. Vis. Sci.,* 1998, 75(6): 388–398.

Smith E.L., Hung L., Harwerth R.S., Effects of optically induced blur on the refractive status of young monkeys. *Vis. Res.,* 1994, 34(3): 293–301.

Smith P.B., Treatment of sight problems by the Bates method: a two year study. 1978, (unpublished).

Smith W., Report on ocular reconditioning. *Am. J. Optom. Arch. Am. Acad. Optom.,* 1945, 22(11): 499–533.

Trachtman J.N., Giambalvo V., The Baltimore myopia study 40 years later. *J. Behav. Optom.,* 1991, 2: 47–50.

Trachtman J.N., Biofeedback of accommodation to reduce functional myopia. *Am. J. Optom. Physiol. Opt.,* 1978, 55(6): 400–406.

Trachtman J.N., Biofeedback of accomodation to reduce myopia, a review. *Am. J. Optom. Physiol. Opt.,* 1987, 64: 639–643.

Treue S., Perceptual enhancement of contrast by attention. *Trends Cog. Sci.,* 2004, 8(10): 435–437.

Troilo D., Wallman J., The regulation of eye growth and refractive state: an experimental study of emmetropization. *Vis. Res.,* 1991, 31(7/8): 1237–1250.

Woo G.C., Wilson M.A., Current methods of treating and preventing myopia. *Optom. Vis. Sci.,* 1990, 67(9): 719–727.

Woods A., Report from the Wilmer Institute on the results obtained in the treatment of myopia by visual training. *Am. J. Ophth.,* 1946, 29(1): 28–57.

Yackle K., Fitzgerald D.E., Emmetropization: an overview. *J. Behav. Optom.,* 1999, 2: 38–43.

Young F.A., The development and control of myopia in human and subhuman primates. *Contacto,* 1975, (19)6: 16–31.

Young F.A., The effect of restricted space on the refractive error of the young monkey eye. *Invest. Ophth.*, 1963, 2: 571–577.

Young F.A., The nature and control of myopia. *J. Am. Optom. Assoc.*, 1977, (48)4: 451–457.

Young F.A., Leary. G.A., Accommodation and vitreous chamber pressure: a proposed mechanism for myopia. In Grosvenor T.G., Flom M.C., eds., *Refractive Anomalies: Research and Clinical Applications*. Butterworth-Heinemann, 1991, 301–309.

Young F.A., Leary. G.A., The inheritance of ocular components. *J. Optom. Arch. Am. Acad. Optom.*, 1972, (49)7: 546–555.

Young F.A., Leary G.A., Baldwin W.R., West D.C., The transmission of refractive errors within Eskimo families. *Am. J. Optom. Arch. Am. Acad. Optom.*, 1969, (46)9: 676–685.

INDEX

Strabismus (Crossed eyes) (*continued*):
    patching for, 39–40, 44, 86
      statistics on, 23
      surgery for, 122
Stress, effects of, 40, 43, 75–77, 97, 99, 112, 183
Stress-relieving lenses, 183
Sunglasses, 43, 137, 152
Sunning, 129, 132
Swinging, 105, 116, 127–128, 132
Syntonics, 26

Tear fluid contact lenses, 187
Therapeutic lenses, 26, 29, 118, 182–183
Thumb fusion, 94
Tone, Franchot, 100
Tossing, 135
Tractional retinal detachment, 175
Traditional eye care, 26, 30, 32, 41, 117, 119, 143–144
Training lenses, 118
Trifocals, 173
20-20-20 rule, 147, 156

UC Berkeley School of Optometry, 122
Ultraviolet (UV) radiation, 24, 151–152, 167

University of Houston, 28

van Vogt, E. A., 100
Viral conjunctivitis, 172
Vision therapy (three phases of), 36–37
Visual cortex, 18, 186
Visual deprivation, 144
Visual system (workings of), 16–17
Vitrectomy, 161, 175
Vitreous gel, 157–158, 160–162, 175

Washington State University, 117
Wet (exudative) macular degeneration, 167
Windolph, Michael, 131
Windolph Technique, 131–132
Worrell, Burton, 122

Yale Clinic of Child Development, 116
Yantras, 97
Yoga, 26, 97, 105
The Yoga Sutras (Pantanjali), 97
Young, Francis, 27, 29, 117, 170, 183–184
Young's Formula, 170, 183–185

Zonule of Zinn, 17–18

ABOUT THE
AUTHORS

Dr. Merrill J. Allen, O.D., Ph.D.

Professor emeritus and former Head of the School of Optometry at Indiana University. During his distinguished career, he educated thousands of optometrists and published 236 research papers and two textbooks.

He conducted seminal research into automobile safety and was responsible for many of the features that have become standard elements of automobile design, including high-mounted tail lights, nonreflective dashboards, and front and rear fender side lights.

Throughout his teaching and research career, Dr. Allen was recognized by academia, government, and private industry as a world expert in vision-related standards and highway safety. In recognition of his achievements, he received numerous honors including the American Optometric Association's Apollo Award and the British Optical Association's Research Medal.

Dr. Steven M. Beresford, Ph.D.

Research scientist with a doctorate in quantum mechanics and electron spin resonance spectroscopy. He was part of the group that developed the original technology that led to magnetic resonance imaging (MRI), which is used in hospitals throughout the world.

During the course of his career, he has served as an associate at the Portland State University Department of Physics where he carried out research into low temperature nuclear fusion, and as a Portland community college professor.

He was instrumental in forming the team of optometrists that carried out research into vision therapy eye exercises, resulting in the techniques used in the Power Vision Program. He has carried out seminal research into the biomechanics of the eyes including enhanced image formation and cataract reversal.

Dr. Francis A. Young, Ph.D.

Professor emeritus and former Head of Washington State University Primate Research Center, which he founded with a building grant from the National Institutes of Health and which currently houses the Environmental Health Services program.

During the course of his career, he carried out seminal research into the cause of myopia, ranging from vision studies of astronauts to the occurrence of myopia in Eskimo (Inuit) children who were being absorbed into the American school system, and the occurrence of myopia in twins and nonhuman primates.

As one of the world's foremost myopia researchers, he published 120 research papers and three texbooks and received numerous honors including the American Optometric Association's Apollo Award and a listing in "Who's Who in the World."

Notes

Notes

Notes

Notes

Notes

Notes

Notes

Notes

Notes

Notes